Yogic Secrets of the Vedas

YOGIC SECRETS OF THE VEDAS

Exploring the Roots of Yoga and Ayurveda

YOGI BABA PREM TOM BEAL

ADITYA PRAKASHAN
New Delhi

ISBN 978-81-7742-102-6

website: www.adityaprakashan.com

Published by Aditya Prakashan, 2/18, Ansari Road, New Delhi – 110 002.
Printed at Rajkamal Electric Press

This book would not be possible without the work, dedication, and blessings from many people. I dedicate this offering to my Guru Mahavatar Babaji, without you I would be lost in the darkness.

To David Frawley (Pandit Vamadeva Shastri), my Vedic teacher, your example is truly a guide to the world. Without your kindness and help it would have been very difficult to connect with these important teachings. Words cannot express my gratitude.

To Dayamata Shakti Prem, when the storm was at its darkest, you were the only one that truly offered help and compassion. You are one of the great souls that serve as a householder on this planet, for the benefit of humanity.

Contents

Preface

In my personal journey of spirituality, after 25+ years of dedication and study, I have come to realize that within the perfection of the cosmos every step, every challenge, every opportunity was a result of my karma, blessings from God and Guru and as a preparation for the study of Vedic yoga.

It can only be assumed that if you have found an attraction, interest, or casual glance at this book that your karmas are affording you an opportunity to grow closer to your personal time of deepening study and realization.

It is a tremendous blessing, opportunity, and task to develop a serious study of spiritual principles. But in reality that is the purpose of life. All other issues are merely an opportunity to come closer to spiritual study, or to resolve karma in order to approach the spiritual path in a future incarnation. Either way spirituality walks with each of us every moment of every day. Today I will secretly celebrate with you the beginning of this journey towards Vedic Yoga.

My personal journey towards writing this book is one that required over 25 years of meditation, study and practice. It seriously began in the late 1980s, after my kundalini first awoke. Working with the kundalini energy guided me toward the study of Sanskrit and ultimately the Vedas. In the initial years, virtually everyone told me that the study of Sanskrit and the Vedas was a waste of time. But yet, some unseen force, desire, maybe a longing continued to inspire me towards this study.

After years of searching, experiencing rejection at every turn, I found Pandit Vamadeva Shastri (Dr. David Frawley). When we met, at his home in Santa Fe, New Mexico, I explained my desire to study the Vedas and lack of support from the yogic community and teachers. He calmly smiled, and we began a journey that would expand my spiritual understanding and provide a solid system of communication for fundamental communication of the mystical experience.

Often the mystical experience is difficult to describe; as the limitations of language are often revealed when discussing the mystical realms. Regrettably, this has resulted in religion moving away from the mystical experience, or even valuing the mystical experience at times. Our lack of clear communication of the mystical experience has resulted in humanity slowly losing our understanding of the deep mystical states left by our forefathers, ancestors and saints.

As new mystics have emerged over the past 100 years, they have attempted to create a new mystical language, but this has resulted in much confusion amongst students of different teachers. The Vedas and mystical teachings of the Vedas provide a unifying form of communication in regards to communication of mystical experience. Additionally, the Vedic deities represent universal concepts, truths and teachings. Understanding the Vedic deity, their role and function, has much to offer the modern study of religion, spirituality and mysticism. While modern society, especially the western world, has moved away from terms such as mysticism; this is primarily due to the propagation of falsehoods and incorrect information by religious zealots.

The purpose of this book is to introduce the modern world to Vedic Yoga. As Vedic Yoga is probably the oldest form of yoga currently known to humanity; it is also the least know. It is most likely the mother of all yoga systems. Within the Vedic yoga tradition, I found a comprehensive system that was extremely practical for the modern day student of yoga and spirituality. Additionally, I discovered a system that addressed many of the common day problems and challenges of our society. Vedic yoga offers important teachings and solutions for our current age. It also has the ability, as with all yoga systems, to meet the student at their current level of consciousness and gently begin to elevate them to higher levels of consciousness and realization. It also seems like our current age needs this information that the Vedic teachings have so carefully preserved over untold millenia. I feel it has been one of the greatest blessings in my heart to have had the opportunity to learn from and experience the Vedic teachings.

It is important to note that this book would not have been possible without the nurturing guidance of Pandit Vamadeva Shastri (Dr. David Frawley). He has tireless served the world by providing some of the most important work on Vedic teachings, inspiring scholars globally; but more importantly, I find that he is the embodiment of the Vedic tradition comprising the important areas of kindness, generosity and knowledge. Over four decades of his life has been dedicated to sharing Vedic knowledge globally. His books are some of the most accessible and informative on Vedic subjects such as Ayurveda, Vedic yoga and Vedic astrology. Without his dedication, guidance and assistance, this book could have never have come into being.

Foreword

Yoga is the essence of Vedic philosophy, which aims at the unification of the human being with the greater conscious universe. Yoga, one could say, is the Vedic way of action, arising from the Vedic understanding of One Self and Being pervading all beings and becomings. The specific term Yoga first arises in the mantras of the Rig-veda where it speaks of Yoga or yoking the higher intelligence (dhi) for the purposes of uniting us with the higher light of truth. However, many other aspects of Yoga and various synonyms for Yoga abound in Vedic texts, including commonly known yogic terms like *mantra*, *dhyana* (meditation), *karma*, *dharma*, *prana* and *tapas*. We should not reduce the spectrum of concerns associated with Yoga to a single term, even the word Yoga. In fact, the Vedas themselves are a path of Mantra Yoga that itself encompasses all the other Yoga paths of knowledge, devotion and works, including physical and psychological techniques, such as we find extending into later Vedanta and Tantra.

Yoga, which is hidden in the Vedic mantras, is first clearly defined in the Upanishads (note, for example, Svetasvatara IV), the great spiritual scriptures of ancient India, in terms of Vedic deities of Agni, Soma, Vayu and Surya, the great powers of Fire, Moon, Wind and Sun, not as external luminaries but as lights of awareness, which is their inner meaning in the Vedas themselves. Yoga is defined in the Bhagavad Gita (Chapter IV) as an inner type of Vedic yajna or sacrifice, reflecting the inner yogic meaning of all Vedic rituals as offerings to the Divine within, which also exist in the earliest Vedic mantras as well.

In the outer Vedic sacrifice, there are three main priests, the *hota* who invokes the deities with the mantras, the *adhvaryu* who makes the offerings, and the *udgata* who performs the closing singing and praise. These three priests are identified with the Vedic deities of *Agni* (Fire), *Vayu* (Air) and *Surya* (Sun). At an inner level, Agni is said to be speech and the *hota*, *Vayu* is said to be the mind and the *adhvaryu*, and *Surya* is said to be *prana* and the *udgata*.

The inner Vedic sacrifice consists of offering speech, mind and *prana*, what could be called our 'inner priests' or guiding faculties, into the light of the indwelling Self. This forms the basis for the practices of mantra yoga, *pranayama* or *prana* yoga and meditation (dhyana yoga), the yoga of the mind. While the Vedic approach can be more complex and many sided than this simple formulation, with other variations and expansions on these basic correlations, this orientation should serve to provide the reader with a good idea of the inner Vedic focus. All that we see in nature is also a force within our own psyche and a power of Yoga or union with all.

Unfortunately, few scholars or even yoga teachers, particularly in the West, have bothered to look into, much less discover the Vedic roots of Yoga, even though these are not difficult to trace for one who makes the effort. What is required is a knowledge of the Vedic language and a sensitive mind to the meaning of Vedic symbols. Above all, one must be a practitioner of the Vedic teachings or their inner meanings cannot unfold. The Vedic texts teach karma yoga or the yoga of service and ritual at an outer level, which itself is quite sophisticated and complex. The Vedic texts themselves, composed of mantras represent mantra yoga at an inner level. Vedic mantras, like the *Gayatri* which is still widely used as an aid to meditation by millions of seekers world wide, are not only mantra yoga but use mantra to promote knowledge and devotion as well. Mantra itself is the inner vehicle of all the Yogas.

The Vedic hymns honor the Divine in the form of various Gods and Goddesses throughout all of nature, and in terms of all main human associations as father, mother, brother, sister, master, beloved and friend. This worship, which is not only outer but also inner, provides the foundation of Bhakti Yoga or the Yoga of devotion, which is the main Yoga of the Rig veda in its many hymns of praise (Suktas) to the Divine as Thou or the main object of our adoration. Jnana Yoga or the Yoga of knowledge and Self-realization is more difficult to find clearly delineated in Vedic texts but commonly occurs hidden in the symbolism of many mantras, particularly the Vedic idea of searching out the supreme Agni or original light of truth in the spiritual heart in which the entire universe dwells. Surya or the Sun reflects the light of the Atman, and Indra or the Supreme Deity of the Vedas, indicates the light of direct perception. Soma, the Vedic nectar, itself at an inner level is the *ananda* or *amrit* from the meditative mind of the crown *chakra* or *Sahasrara*.

Yogi Baba Prem is one of the few western yoga teachers who has taken the time and applied the energy to look into the Vedic origins of Yoga and delve into what the Vedic Yoga was likely to have been, as well as those intimations of its practices that still remain. He has made the considerable effort both to learn the Vedic Sanskrit, which is even more difficult than classical Sanskrit, and to uncover the yogic secrets of the Vedic symbolism, which can be quite arcane given the great antiquity of the Vedic teaching that reflects an earlier world age or *yuga* and its very different language and minset.

His book 'Yogic Secrets of the Vedas' provides a number keys to the yogic meaning of the Vedic deities and indicates several primary Vedic yogic approaches in detail. Such a deeper approach to the Vedic Yoga opens new ground for scholars and spiritual seekers alike: for scholars to take off their blinders and face the depth of Vedic mysticism and for seekers so that they can employ at least a few Vedic practices in a meaningful and contemporary manner. Vedic deities like Indra, Agni and Ushas come alive for his readers and began to move and spiritual forces within us under his inspiration.

I have known Baba Prem for many years now and have seen his many insightful articles and books on Yoga, Ayurveda, Veda and Tantra. I have seen the important research that he is selflessly conducting and have encouraged him to publish it. In this regard he moves in the line of scholars more in the Vedic tradition and in lines of great modern gurus like Sri Aurobindo and Kavyakantha Ganapati Muni. India often provides a more fertile ground for sharing such deeper studies, as I myself have discovered with my own work, so it is good to see his work presented to the Indian audience as well.

Such work on the Vedic Yoga as he has done is necessary today to help us reclaim our global spiritual heritage. It helps link us once more to the wisdom of our ancient spiritual ancestors that we desperately need to move out of our current global crisis, caught as we are between the two evils of commercialism and religious fundamentalism that are literally destroying our planet tearing the human psyche apart as well as the Vedas restore our living link to the sacred universe that no church, government or business can own or represent.

It is my hope that the book will gain a good readership among serious practitioners and dedicated seekers, as well as open minded and intuitive scholars. Yoga students and teachers in India should look at the book to see that knowledge of the Vedic Yoga is again rising in the Western world, which they are used to, in the line of Max Mueller, seeing only the outer face of the Vedas and missing the inner heart. Such studies can help stimulate them to conduct similar research of their own.

A yogic renaissance is necessary today, with new insightful approaches to yogic teachings, not so much for the body but for the higher mind and spiritual heart. The Vedas provide the mantric key to that highest endeavor of humanity to return to Unity. The writings of Yogi Baba Prem help lead us in that direction as well.

Dr. David Frawley (Pandit Vamadeva Shastri)
Director, American Institute of Vedic Studies
Santa Fe, New Mexico
May 2010

Introduction

For untold millennia, mankind has struggled with its history, heritage, and lineage of knowledge. Within modern history, we have seen a great distortion of its secret truths. Regrettably, the record of history will always contain a cultural predisposition or bias. And apparently, history will always be recorded from the perspective of the victor or dominant group. This ultimately results in a great distortion of a plethora of subjects, histories, and religions. While it would be correct to say that many valiant souls have struggled to maintain a precise record of the known history of humanity, in reality very few laymen have the opportunity to explore the vast amount of information currently archived within modern academia. In fact, few scholars have the time to wade through the copious volumes of recorded information. Within the view of world history the distortion of facts appears no stronger than within religion and spirituality.

The distortion of religious teachings and history has a shaded history with drama that would rival any modern movie or book. It is filled with violence, political agendas, deception, greed, lust for power, and other qualities that we as a society currently value in fiction writings. Within India's Vedic tradition, we find blatant examples of distorting historical teachings and facts by external groups. Additionally, we find that the purity of the ancient teachings of yoga have been colored by western scholars; while noble in their scholarly pursuits have sometimes missed the forest for the trees.

My personal journey, towards the Vedas and to literally experience the **Yogic Secrets of the Vedas**, began with the study of yoga and my own personal *Kundalini* awakening experience in the mid 1980's. As I learned to work with the *Kundalini* energy, I found myself drawn to Sanskrit initially, and this led to a powerful attraction towards the Vedas. Most teachers that I encountered had little or no knowledge of Sanskrit, or of the Vedas. In fact, I had to teach myself basic Sanskrit with the aid of home study courses and a powerful desire to learn more about the Vedas. Once my initial basic study of Sanskrit was complete, I sought out information on the Vedas. It was difficult to find quality information on the Vedas, and the naturalistic interpretations from the late 1800's were quite prevalent. I would meet with western teachers and express my desire to study the Vedas, only to be greeted with a bewildered look and most commonly the question, "Why?" It was difficult to answer, their question. I did not know enough about the Vedas to even know why. But at the same time, I could not resist the powerful impulse to learn about the Vedas. It seemed, intuitively to me, that great secrets were contained within it. Possibly, the Vedas contained solutions to the world's challenges, or a knowledge or technology that the world was in need of.

My search continued for many years. I was becoming familiar with the work of Dr. David Frawley (Pandit Vamadeva Shastri). He, at the time, had written several books on the Vedas and Vedic teachings. These books seemed to "feed the need" that my mind called out for. I eventually had the opportunity meet him in the United States, and discussed how no one could support my desire to study the Vedas. He just smiled, but also proceeded to guide my Vedic study over the next decade; teaching me about select vedangas and upavedas, and nurturing my study of the Vedas itself. It is through this process, that this book is even possible.

Eventually, I received the titles of Veda Kovid for proficiency with the Vedas, and then the traditional title of Veda Visharada meaning a more comprehensive knowledge of the Vedas.

Pandit Vamadeva Shastri's work has ignited a reawakening to the Vedic teachings and in particular Vedic yoga. This is important as the Vedas serve as the mother of all yoga systems. Regrettably, few yoga teachers focus on the Vedas or the important teachings they contain, and a great deal of confusion exists regarding the Vedas to this very day. It is my hope that this book will open the way for the reader to experience a small portion of the Vedic concepts and teachings; possibly opening the door towards greater realization and understanding, practical application of Vedic knowledge in their daily life, as well as their sadhana. The Vedas are amongst the most practical spiritual teachings I have ever encountered. Providing a deep spiritual teaching that is steeped in practical application, as-well-as deep mystical insight into the nature of humanity and their relationship with divinity.

The History of Vedic Yoga

While it is true that Vedic yoga is relatively unknown to most modern practitioners of yoga, it does serve as the root and foundation for most other known yoga systems. To understand Vedic yoga, one must travel back in time to the north central and northwestern regions of India. This is the motherland of Vedic yoga, and the homeland of the Vedic civilization and culture.

A great deal of information is being discovered about this ancient civilization through study of ancient texts, archaeological evidence and satellite imagery. While it was long believed that this ancient culture was an invading race from a distant land, known as the "Aryan" race; the evidence simply does not support this hypothesis. In reality, the Vedic people of this region were the "Aryans"[1] which were divided into several lineages of people. The most common known today were the Nahusha people, which were divided into 5 different groups, occupying different parts of the Vedic homeland. If one were to refer to the Aryan race it would be a reference to these people and a few groups that were older. What is more important is the concept of Aryan culture. The term "Aryan Culture" transcends race and social/ economic groups which define countries today.

The evidence of a Vedic culture is voluminous and displays an ancient world that was extremely mobile and well traveled. Within the *Vayu Purana*[2] examples are given to the depth and

[1]Aryan is a Sanskrit term that means noble.

[2]The *Vayu Purana* is one of the oldest puranas known to humanity. Puranas consist of what is called remembered information. It is information that has been traditionally handed down over long periods of time.

size of the Vedic culture. There are numerous references to 7 continents, seven oceans, and subcontinents. More importantly there is a reference to the Vedic lands as being quite expansive and surrounded by salt-water seas on all sides, suggesting that the Vedic Aryans considered all of Europe, Asia, and Asia Minor to be part of the Vedic culture.

Mummies found in China, circa 1906, were discovered to not resemble people from the Orient, but rather had numerous European features and characteristics; including, but not limited to blond and most importantly red colored hair. Science has suggested a migration of European peoples to this region, but it is possible that these were travelers and visitors to portions of the Vedic culture, possibly returning for a sacred ritual, or a type of pilgrimage.

The age of the Vedic civilization is not clearly known, as the Hindu system deals with time periods that were inconceivable to western minds until relatively recently. It would clearly be safe to say that the Vedic teachings go back to the end of the last ice age, circa 8000 BCE. Within the Rig Veda, we find astrological references dating to about 6500 BCE. So one can be confident that Vedic Yoga is at least 8500 years old, with the reality being that it is most likely considerably older, as it is not realistic to believe that these teachings suddenly manifested in a short period of time.

While many accounts present people of this age as in backward, primitive people, the reality is that they were a spirituality-advanced group that valued "animism". Whereas animism is devalued in our present society, it was in reality not a purely naturalistic, frightened religious system as is presented by many scholars. It was a common and basic belief that all of nature was divine. That divinity permeated all aspects of life and every manifestation of life. This is the foundation of most "New-Age" beliefs in modern society. It is also reflected in a variety of teachings such as the Native American tradition. It even appears in Christianity with terms such as omnipotent, though the Church does not heavily focus on this concept.

Vedic yoga is one of the, if not the oldest spiritual system known to mankind. The reality is that all people practice some form of spirituality from Vedic yoga, even if they are not aware of the proper term. As Vedic yoga appears to be the only record we have of the original mother of all yoga and spiritual systems.

The Vedic Link with other Yoga Systems

While most people do not recognize the Vedic link with other yoga systems, with study it becomes quite apparent. While the *Rig Veda* is clearly the oldest book known to mankind that is still used to this day. Most people do not realize that it is a *samhita*, which is a work that refers to mantra only. As a *samhita*, the Vedas contain primarily mantras; these mantras were revealed while rishis were in deep meditation.

Within Vedic yoga, the primary techniques consist of:

1. Mantra. (Repetition of sacred sounds)
2. Pranayama. (Control of the breath)
3. Dhyana. (Meditation)
4. Yajna. (offerings)

We will explore these later; first let's examine Vedic yoga's connection with other yoga systems.

The Yoga Sutras of Patanjali and their Vedic Link

Probably the most influential yogic teaching on modern society would be the "Yoga Sutras of Patanjali". Most yoga teachers and many students of yoga have at least been introduced to this work. While many can quote from this book, which is an accomplishment in the west, it is seldom that anyone explores beyond basic commentaries on the yoga sutras, and fewer recognize its roots within the Vedic tradition.

Patanjali the writer

Virtually nothing seems to be known about Patanjali — the man. In some stories, he is the son of Brahman, in others he is born on Mount Meru. In India, Mount Meru is the sacred mountain. It is 350,000 miles in size, and is surrounded by 7 continents. Obviously, this is a reference to the spinal column and the nadis (streams of energy) of the body, which total 350,000. The 7 continents are a reference to the primary chakas. He is also considered to have written the text *Mahabhasya.* The Mahabhasya took Panini's 4000 laws of Sanskrit grammar to another level in terms of organization and systematic codification. His authorship of this may be true or not true. In India, there is a growing opinion that he also wrote under the name Charaka, and was responsible for the Charaka Samhita, a major Ayurvedic text[1]. It has also been thought that possibly numerous writers wrote under his name.

Patanjali was considered by some to be an incarnation of Ananta. Ananta was the thousand headed ruler of the serpent race. This statement alone could have numerous implications from being a reference to the Kundalini, to such groups as the Nagas. The dates of his life are not truly known, but it is believed that he lived circa 200 BCE. The *Yoga Sutras* are believed to have been recorded around 100-200 CE according to modern scholars.

It seems possible that Patanjali was most certainly a skilled teacher and obviously skilled in Vedic teachings, as will be explored later. It is quite possible that Patanjali's compilation was created circa 200 BCE and later recorded between 100-200 CE as humanity continued moving away from the previous world age. There is some evidence to support this hypothesis, and this was a common occurrence with ancient teachings; as they were commonly preserved in a verbal or oral tradition, eventually being recorded in written form at a much later date.

The Vedas themselves were preserved in an oral tradition, moving to a more exclusive written form near the end of the Vedic period circa 1800 BCE. Clearly, the evidence supports

---

[1]Ayurveda is an ancient healing system. It is considered an upaveda or secondary Vedas making it part of the Vedic system of teachings. Ayurveda consists of herbs, lifestyle practices, mantra, and yajnas to promote balance and a healthy lifestyle.

the Vedic teachings as being much older than the period that they were compiled in their present form. Likewise, it is quite possible that the same was true for Patanjali also.

What is most profound is the appearance of an invocation to Patanjali. The invocation to Patanjali appears almost 800-900 years later in commentaries recorded by a king known as Bhoja. This work is commonly referred to as the *Vritti Bhoja*, literally meaning Bhoja's thoughts. What is most interesting is that usually this implies a lineage. Likewise, it is interesting to note the length between the writing by Patanjali and appearance of later commentaries regarding the "Yoga Sutras". It is traditional to invoke the founder or current master of a particular lineage. It seems quite possible that Patanjali could have taught in a secret lineage; whose teachings remained quite secret until the need to record the information became evident due to concerns over information becoming lost. As previously mentioned, this theory would fit with the other traditional models observed within India. It is most interesting that a well-known type of Hatha yoga still uses the invocation of Patanjali; though few seem to truly realize that they are invoking an ancient lineage that was quite comfortable with the Vedic tradition.

Patanjali's Vedic Connection

Regardless of the date of Patanjali, he would have missed such times as the India medieval period, the Muslim Invasions, or the British occupation. It is difficult to believe that he did not participate in Vedic traditions to some degree. Most writers suggest that Patanjali's compilation of the Yoga Sutras marked a difference between the Vedic Yoga and what we currently know as yoga. Some writers state that Patanjali's yoga was dualistic. This is difficult to believe in light that the Purusha occupies the highest state within the "Yoga Sutras", being the untouched observer. But in reality, there is little evidence to support this statement pertaining to the dualistic approach of Patanjali.

In some traditions, it was believed that Patanjali was strongly connected with Shaivism, possibly even a Shaivite master. While one could look at this tradition, we do find some evidence to support it. Based on the thirty six tattvas of the Shivite tradition, Purusha would function as a lower manifestation of limited consciousness, a reflection of the higher consciousness (Shiva) supporting the idea of dualism. But this seems to be a weak theory, as Patanjali in the sutras is clear regarding the superior state of Purusha. But yet, we see evidence of terms within the "Yoga Sutras" that are clearly from the Vedic/Vedantic traditions.

What is most interesting, and clearly demonstrates a Vedic connection is the word Brahmacharya. Brahmacharya appears within the first limb of the sutras. It is commonly taught as celibacy. While there can be little argument as to this meaning, is there more to the word than this? Brahmacharya comes from two roots: Brahma and Charya. Brahma is a reference to the Vedic Brahman, and Charya means conduct. Brahmacharya would literally mean conduct of a Brahman. The verbal roots for charya is *car* meaning to move and the root for brahman being *brh* meaning to make strong (Commonly the interpretation would be celibacy. While celibacy would fulfill this, it also seems that other interpretations would also need to be considered.) This could also refer to Vedic activities such as the Vedic ritual albeit internal or external. It would appear that Patanjali was referring both. It is also the mind moving toward oneness with Brahman. Brahmacharya also refers to the conduct of a student while studying *Brahma Vidya* or Vedic knowledge. What is Brahma Vidya, if not the mind moving toward oneness with the source of all — Brahman. It seems strange that Patanjali would select such a word as this unless there was a link between yoga and the Vedic system.

It is possible that the primary focus is Brahma Vidya in which the other limbs are tools for obtaining, or the entire yoga sutras should focus on Brahma Vidya. Just as some scholars feel the entire book is written to address the second sutra, the entire book addresses the older teachings of Brahma Vidya. If the code of conduct for study of Brahma vidya is present, it only seems logical that the study of Brahma Vidya would be a part of it also. It seems that in its higher form the yoga sutras should prepare, involve, and evolve into the study of Brahma Vidya. Since Patanjali only recorded information and was not the source, and used Vedic and Vedantic terms, it seems difficult to omit this from teachings of the yoga sutras, though this has clearly been done. But are there any other teachings to support the more expansive view of Brahmacharya? Yes!

Within the *Darshana Upanishad* is an explanation of Brahmacharya meaning the mind's movement toward Brahman. The Darshan Upanishad is patterned after the "Yoga Sutras"; it does have connections with Vedanta or yoga teachings based in Vedanta. Written by Dattaatreya, he was considered an incarnation of Vishnu and is believed to be the author of the important Advaitic work "Tripura Rahasya" and other works, making him an important writer in Vedanta or more correctly Advaita Vedanta.

There are other terms Patanjali used that are rooted in Vedic/ Vedantic teachings such as:

Purusha.
Prakriti.
The gunas.
Tapas.
Japa and many others.

Bhakti and its place in the Yoga Sutras

Often the Yoga Sutras are criticized for not having the teachings of Bhakti within them. It is believed that they are somehow not Vedic based due to this lack of Bhakti. This is often due to a lack of understanding on the part of the practitioner. Often, this is due to the practitioner not being exposed to the older commentaries pertaining to the Yoga Sutras such as the "Vritti Bhoja" or the commentaries by Vyasas. Even a quick examination of these texts will reveal the existence and firm establishment of Bhakti within the "Yoga Sutras".

Within the Niymas, the 5th practice is ãívarpraçidhanàá va or surrender to God. While terms such as Purusha are often used, this is not to be construed as different from God in a non-dualistic system or even a qualified non-dualistic system. This is evident again with such teachers of ashtanga Yoga, such as Yamunacaarya and Nathamuni; who were clearly practitioners of Bhakti. Even Dattreya, meaning son of Atri, would have been a practitioner of Bhakti. To say that Bhakti does not exist would be such as outrageous a claim as if one was saying that Ramana Maharishi did not believe in Bhakti. Other examples of the practice of Bhakti within the "Yoga Sutras" would be:

> "Or concentrating on the supreme blissful light." I. 36.
> "Or devotion dedicated to the Supreme God (Ishvara)." I. 23.
> "Ishvara is the Purusha..." I. 24.
> "Within him is the seed of omniscience and its complete manifestation." I. 25.
> "Unconditioned by time, He is the teacher of the ancients." I.26 (referring to Ishvara.)
> "Samadhi is attained by surrender to God." II. 45.
> "Spiritual Study brings communion with the personal deity." II. 44.

Yet with all these references to Ishvara, it is not difficult to find the teaching of Bhakti; which has all but disappeared within the teaching of the "Yoga Sutras" in the modern world.

Conclusion

The key seems to rest in the realization that the "Yoga Sutras of Patanjali" have never been intended to exist without a commentary. The role of the commentary is to introduce the student to higher awareness and inferred knowledge that is intended to accompany them. That is why they are written in sutra form. It must be remembered that a sutra is the bare essential information for ease of memorization, and contains a rich body of information behind it in order to complete the teaching itself. I have tried to illustrate this with just a few examples such as Bhakti and Brahmacharya. This same process is clearly illustrated in the monumental work by Jai Deva Singh in the "Shiva Sutras". His important work includes sutras and detailed information that was to accompany each sutra. Clearly, this would have been the case in the time of Patanjali also. Additional commentaries do exist, but most modern students are never exposed to even the slightest mention of these additional commentaries.

Patanjali was the complier of the yoga sutras, which clearly indicates that he was drawing on older, more established teachings. Terms such as Brahmacharya, japa, tapas, Purusha, Ishvara, among others, clearly point to the Vedic roots of his compilation. It is my opinion that the "Yoga Sutras of Patanjali" were not to be separate from the Vedic teachings, but were an important preparatory step from the yogic tradition. The eight limbs prepare the mind and body for the more esoteric stages of spiritual awareness presented in Vedanta and the Vedas themselves. It is a natural course for many students to eventually evolve into the study of the Vedic system. This would most likely begin with the study of the "Bhagavad Gita" as it is a perfect and powerful introduction to the Vedic teachings, offering practical and esoteric information about the nature of existence and spiritual realization. Whereas Patanjali was the compiler of the Yoga sutras, Krishna in "The Bhagavad Gita" states that he was the giver of yoga.

Imaṁ vivasvate yogaṁ proktavān aham avyayam
Vivasvān manave prātha manur ikṣvākave bravīt

Evaṁ paramparāprāptam imaṁ rājaṛṣayo viduḥ
Sa kāleneha mahatā yogo naṣṭaḥ paraṁtapa
—Bhagavad Gita 4.1-2

Here Krishna states, and I paraphrase, that he gave yoga to the sun god and that it was passed to Manu, and to the Ishvaku, coming to the rajarishis and that it was lost over time.

While the date of the *Bhagavad Gita* (commonly referred to as the Gita) is not known for sure, it could have been 5 BCE, though I have seen scholars post dates between 2000-1000 BCE. Much research is being conducted, and the dates for the Bhagavad Gita seem to be being pushed back even further. Using information from the Puranas clearly puts the dates back to an earlier period. It is possible that Patanjali recognized that the ancient teachings were becoming lost again and his attempt to compile them was based on Krishna's teaching in the Gita. Ironically, it is possible that his compilation has only furthered the loss of information unless students accept the task and begin exploring his sutras more deeply, and allow the yoga sutras to inspire them to seeking out higher levels of knowledge, which may have been its purpose anyway.[2]

Analyzing the Sutras

It is quite obvious that modern studies have not focused with the same intensity on the ancient teachings as the ancient writers have. There are numerous reasons for this:

1) The deeper teachings have not been taught openly and on occasion are not suitable for the masses. Often yoga students remain at a relative beginner level of yoga practice, or focus primarily on asana only. This is often due to family, school, career, and social obligations, which limit study and practice time. This has also become true with yoga teachers. Very few have the time or opportunity for in-depth study.
2) Language barriers of Sanskrit — Sanskrit is an extremely complex language, especially in its Vedic form. Few students have the time, depth, and knowledge to explore the beauty, depth, and secrets hidden within the Sanskrit language. To explore this more, let's examine a few Sanskrit words and one sutra from *The Yoga Sutras of Patanjali*.

---

[2] Sources, References and Suggested Reading:

Examination of Dhyana

Roots of the word Dhyana

The Sanskrit word for meditation is Dhyana, which comes from the verbal root dhi or dhya. Both roots mean to "think", this is particularly true in the sense of inquiry, examination or introspection. In fact, in Vedic yoga, "dhi" is a reference to the Buddhi or thinking and discerning mechanism of the mind. It would be correct to call the intellect the Buddhi in its lower function. Dhyana as meditation is not merely a quiet mind, though this can be a significant achievement.

One of the initial goals of Dhyana should be proper or controlled thought, clearly illustrated in Patanjali's yoga sutras, which states in the eight limbs that before meditation can begin one must possess concentration (*Dharana*). Concentration is not the removal of thought but the focusing of thought onto a single object or a single thought. An advanced state of the final three limbs (*Dharana*, *Dhyana*, and *Samadhi*) is often referred to as "one-pointedness". One-pointedness is the continuous flow of thought, but each thought is in perfect harmony with the preceding thought. In addition, it could be viewed as such intense concentration that there is a merging with the object of concentration. These two points would indicate that the goal is not mere absence of thought, which is beyond reach of most beginner and intermediate students, but a singular or focused thought rooted in powerful concentration. This focused thought actually forms the basis of practical application of Advaitic philosophy, known as inquiry. This system is one of the most advanced philosophical systems from India. But can more light be shed on the process of meditative thinking? Yes! The importance of thought can be clearly illustrated by the word mantra.

Mantra is derived from the verbal root *man*, which means, to "think", and *tra* as a suffix to man, means to 'rescue".

It would also be correct to interpret *tra* as indicating a means or method. Mantra is controlled thinking that actually rescues or saves the mind. What this means, in reality, is to purify the mind and prepare it for more expansive thought.

For most people, the mind could be viewed as a vast sea with a vast storm flowing across it. The thoughts are waves coming from all directions without rhyme or reason. In fact, for most beginners, the focusing of thought can be a considerable challenge. In the preparatory stages of meditation — learning to relax, they feel like a ship trapped at sea in a horrible storm of thought. They wrestle with the thoughts, attempting to harness the wild activity only to experience frustration, after frustration.

Analyzing a Sutra

The second sutra of the *Yoga Sutras of Patanjali* is considered by some to be the most important sutra in the book. "Yogaś Citta Vṛtti Nirodhaḥ" *Yoga Sutras of Patanjali B.1 s.2*, Yoga is restraint of thought in the field of the mind. Here is an apparent paradox and basis for the misunderstanding. Proper thought leads to restraint of thought, or focused thought leads to restraint of thoughts. Incorrectly, this sutra has led some to consider the absence of thought to be the actual teaching, but Patanjali's selection of the word *nirodhah* (restraint) is the key. Regrettably, this has resulted in many scholars thinking that the elimination of thought is the only goal. Especially, since many scholars consider the second sutra to be the most important sutra, and the rest of the book is written to deal with that one issue.

Nirodhah comes from the root *rudh* which means to 'obstruct", the prefix *ni* literally means lowness or downward motions. Nirodhah means not just restraint of thoughts but to obstruct thoughts of lower nature. This would increase thought and concentration of a higher nature. A more practical modern approach would be restraint of thoughts within the field of the ego, and an objective awareness of the thoughts rising from the cosmic mind (Brahman), or as some systems might say merging into pure thought, or pure consciousness. When the mind becomes fully focused on a single object of examination it is able to transcend itself and merge into pure consciousness. So Nirodhah arises from one-pointedness or *ekagra*. It does not arise from a merely blank or unfocused mind. Extreme one-pointedness is Nirodhah, not simply a mind left blank or wandering.

An examination of the remainder of the *Yoga sutras of Patanjali* will reveal that the last three limbs called Dharana, Dhyana, and Samadhi (concentration, meditation, super consciousness) actually contain thought, and work within the field of thought (material creation, mental creation, emotional creation). The initial key is through proper restraint, control and direction of thought. In fact, the Yamas and Niyamas (controls and restraints) introduced in Patanjali's yoga sutras are founded in control of thought; though the goal often taught to students is just control of action. The goal is actually not just control of action, but ultimately this must become control of thought, which results in these lower or negative thoughts being absent from the field of thought.

For the average beginner student, the journey toward true meditation can easily begin with Pranayama. In its more advanced forms, pranayama is actual control of prana; for beginners, it is literally controlling the breath. Careful examination and practice of simple breathing exercises will quickly reveal a meditative truth. The mind is more easily controlled by controlling the breath. As mentioned earlier, the goal is controlled thought. The concentration required for pranayama begins to bring the thinking process under control. In yogic philosophy, the breath is a reflection of the mind and vice versa. So the easiest path for control of the mind is through control of the breath. Once the basics of breath are accomplished, pranayama can have step two added to it — mantra.

In the Vedic Yoga system, Brahmins (priests) used various breathing exercises (pranayama), which are still in use today. The Vedic technique of chanting requires control of the breath. But mantra takes the controlled thinking process to another level. Mantra begins to purify the field of the mind, further preparing for deeper meditation. Repetition (Japa) of mantra over long periods of time has been demonstrated to have powerful healing and clearing effects on the mind. The use of mantra appears in vedangas and upavedas such *Jyotisha*, *Vastu*, and *Ayurveda*. Not to mention the Rig Veda, Atharva Veda, Yajur Veda and the entire Sama Veda contain numerous mantras for these very purposes. In fact, mantra appears within *Brahmanas*, *Arankyas*, *Puranas*, and *Upanishads*. Invocations and specific mantras are used to prepare the mind to think with many of the major Upanishads such as the *Aitareya* and *Taittiriya*. It is quite clear from reviewing the ancient text that a great importance was placed on mantra. According to the ancient teachings, the first gift the cosmos gave to the physical form was the ingoing breath, and with the outgoing breath mantra was manifested on the physical level.

Mantra is one of the most practical forms of yoga practice. It does not require great strength, physical agility, or practice for excessive lengths of time. Long periods of mantra repetition can be very beneficial, provided a student has cultivated their skills and abilities. Initially, mantra can be practiced aloud, after sometime it should be whispered. But the most profound effect on the mind comes from silent repetition of mantra, but this is also requires more skill on the part of the practitioner. *Japa*, the Sanskrit word for repetition, comes from the root *jap*, which means to whisper. It is important to note that in some Indian systems Japa is broken into two primal roots, *Ja* and *Pa*. *Ja* can refer to the mind, or that which is born, and *Pa* can mean to protect. So in some yogic systems, japa can refer to protecting the mind. After sufficient practice and experience with mantra, then the aspirant's mind is prepared for Dhyana.

In the Vedic yoga system, Dhyana can manifest as many forms; one of the most popular is meditation on the physical form of a deity. This powerful and important tool in Vedic meditation is all but ignored in modern society. This is due to numerous reasons such as:

- A lack of understanding of the techniques for working with deities. This is more of an issue in regards to western teachers, as opposed to Hindu teachers.
- Fear of offending people.
- Concerns over conflicting religious views with students.
- The desire of modern teacher is to please students for financial reward among other reasons.

Meditation on a physical form of the deity is a vital second step in the process of self-realization for many students, though some might argue this point, possibly by pointing out that Buddhism does not use deities. It should be noted that deities such as Tara do appear in several forms of Buddhism, and the image of the Buddha is used in almost all, if not all systems of Buddhism. Though the Buddha image is not thought of as a deity, clearly we can see the same process at work as in the Vedic system. It is important to remember that Gautama Buddha did not rebel against Hinduism; as he often referred to his teaching as "Arya Dharma". Gautama rebelled against the emptiness and unawareness that had developed within the Vedic ritual. In fact, the relationship between Hinduism and Tibetan Buddhism has been a fairly close relationship, with even the Dalai Lama agreeing that the roots of Buddhism come from Hinduism. In addition, Tibetan Buddhism has been critical in preserving numerous Hindu texts, philosophies, and works.

The use of a deified image exists even within the Catholic Church with mother Mary representing the Shakti (feminine power) of divinity. Catholics worship daily to a variety of images of Saints and Angels. This is, in reality, the Catholic SP church's recognition of a Hindu principle, as Hinduism is considerably older. After practicing this technique, one would most certainly agree that it is a powerful technique and form of meditation. The appearance of a deity in Bhakti yoga is a very powerful aspect, though there are some forms of Bhakti that are more oriented toward not accepting attributes.

Working with a deity image is a powerful technique that greatly aids in awakening the higher function of the buddhi (it should be noted that mantra facilitates the awakening of the buddhi also). More abstract forms of deity meditation can be used as the skill of the practitioner increases, such as *yantras*, which serve as the body of the deity in the Tantric system, and with mantra, which serves as the mind of the deity. And still even more advanced meditation can be practiced on the deity by performing samyama on various attributes of the deity and ignoring the form completely; eventually leading to formless meditation for some practitioners that desire to explore that direction. Though some may choose to stay within the field of form, which is a completely valid system too. It is quite clear that the use of a deity image or image for spiritual growth is almost universal. In reality, and with proper education, there should be no conflict with using an image in meditation. It is one of the oldest and most common techniques.

Tantric Roots to the Vedas

While the Tantric system has often been viewed as a later development within the greater field of Hinduism; a deeper study reveals that the roots to Tantric teachings exist within the Vedas themselves. Tantric teachings are based in and are as old as the Vedas itself, representing another side of the Vedic approach.

It is not realistic to expect the Vedas to contain the entire teachings of the Vedic period, but rather as samhitas they contain the *shrutti* or revelations that were given during deep meditation. This point cannot be argued, but it is important to note that there were different schools of Vedic thought and teaching. According to Patanjali in the *Mahabhasya*, there were about 100 different schools of thought pertaining to just the Yajur Veda. While this can be seen as a weakness, it is in reality the strength of Hinduism. By the acceptance of different schools of thought, a comprehensive system of thought and teaching is preserved. While very few schools of thought are preserved today, each one still retains its relevance, importance, and contribution. Westerns scholars made the mistake of assuming that Yaska and particularly Sayana were the final authorities on Vedic subjects, though they only provided a nature oriented view of the Vedas. It is important that the modern student not become dogmatic about different schools of interpretation. Possibly all, or many of the schools were correct in their Vedic approach and interpretation. This broader view makes the Vedas the most powerful and important teaching within humanity.

While scholars have often viewed the Vedas as primarily masculine, the feminine is represented by the Sanskrit letters themselves. There are many Vedic Goddesses like Ila, Ushas, Aditi, and Sarasvati to name just a few. But most importantly and often overlooked is Apas. While apas is viewed as the primordial waters, it is often given a neuter position within the Sanskrit language. But within the *Shatapatha Brahmana (II.1.1.13)*, it clearly states that "[the] waters [apo] are female, Agni is male. This message is repeated in II.1.1.14. In this context, the waters (apas) serve as the shakti of agni, or at a minimum the flow and movement of agni. Within the ritualistic teachings of the Yajur Veda, this relationship between the waters and Agni is very important. On the inner level, the same teaching is reflected within the Rig Veda as the destruction of Vrtra (ego), and the releasing of the waters (knowledge). Apas has a verbal root of *ap*, which means "to obtain". The releasing of the waters is the obtaining or acquiring the realization or experience of Agni. This is reflected through the Tantric practice of merging the masculine and feminine principles together.

Within the *Shatapatha Brahmana (I.1),* it is stated that *svaha* is the feminine form of Agni, or more correctly the opposite polarity in the Vedic ritual. This is why all Vedic fire rituals often contain the word svaha as the offering is being made. This is certainly true with the Agnihotra ceremony. Svaha, personified, is the wife of Agni; the fire ritual cannot be complete without this male/female polarity being present. She also represents the spoken offering as well as the ashes, the transformed matter at the end of the fire ceremony. Again, she is the Shakti of Agni on the inner and the outer level of our being.

The word svaha comes from two words: 1) *su* meaning to move or go, to press out, but more correctly to enliven, impel, or generate. 2) *aha* meaning to say, speak. Together, they enliven speech, generate through speech, or are using speech to impel. It can also mean to press out through speech, and is associated with speech; therefore, Agni and Svaha have a male/female balance with speech.

Within the Vedic Vedi, or fire pit, the same concept is present. We see the fire pit symbolically representing the female energy, and the offering of ghee or other materials as the masculine principle. This foundation of Vedic teaching is another example of the Vedic representation of Tantric principles.

Some temples within India exhibit male and female deities in a physical (sexual) embrace, on the outer walls, while this does not literally refer to sexual Tantra as is often assumed that it does; it again conveys the importance of the Vedic and Tantric teaching of male and female balancing principles. This principle manifests even on the grossest level of manifestation as the female genitalia forming the shape of a flame.

Clearly it can be seen that numerous Tantric principles are rooted from the Vedic teachings. Even the left handed or sexual path of Tantra is rooted within Vedic principles. Regrettably, the sexual aspect of the left-handed path receives the most focus in modern society, and the deep spiritual principles often become obscured.

But do the Tantras refer directly to any of the Vedic deities? The answer is YES!

- Paramananda Tantra 11.35 Surya, Agni and soma are mentioned.
- Gautamiya Tantra mentioned Antar yajna.
- The Shaktisangamatantra mentioned Indra, Chandra, and Manu.
- The Agamas continue or contain the symbolism of the Vedas.
- The Mahanirvanatantra alludes that the agama approach is in harmony with the Vedas.
- The Tantras did teach Antar Yajna, a Vedic principle.

Do more modern sages support this belief and link between Tantra and Vedic teachings; the answer is YES.

- Sri Aurobindo discussed the connection between the Tantras and Vedas.

- T.V. Kapali Shastry also believed that there was a connection between Tantric tradition and the Vedas. Though he acknowledged that they approached the teachings differently. He did believe that they supported the authority of the Vedas.
- Swami Vivekananda supported a connection between the Vedas and Tantras.
- Sri Ramana Maharishi referred to Brahman, terms such as tat tvam asi. He also mentioned that the techniques of Tantra were good for purifying the mind. He actually agreed that most yoga techniques were good for purifying the mind.
- Ganapati Muni (Ramana's disciple) wrote on the connection between the Vedas and Tantra.
- In more modern times, this work has been continued by Pandit Vamadeva Shastri (David Frawley) especially in his book *Tantra Yoga and the Wisdom Goddesses.*

The change in deities within the Tantric system is not in conflict with Vedic teachings, but is more likely a later transition of teachings, just as the Puranas are a later modification and/or memory of original Vedic teachings. Looking within the Vedas as revelation, one can clearly see that most systems of India are rooted within the Vedic teachings and are included within the Tantric system.

Kundalini Yoga and its Vedic Connection

The term '*Kundalini*' is becoming a familiar term amongst students of yoga, but few people are introduced to the depth and breadth of knowledge of this ancient system. Even fewer are familiar with the Vedic roots of Kundalini yoga.

Within Hinduism (*Sanatana Dharma* — eternal teachings), all teachings defer to the spiritual authority of the Vedas. The Vedas are a series of ancient teachings of which the Rig Veda is considered the oldest. While the Vedas has become an obscure text to the general public, it is filled with powerful spiritual teachings and continues to have much relevance to this day.

What the western scholar does not understand, is that the Vedas can be interpreted in a variety of ways, and its meanings are multi-dimensional. From the Hindu viewpoint, all truth must be founded or substantiated with the Vedas; or at minimum, the Vedas is the final authority on spiritual matters. Within the Vedas is hidden a science and understanding of the Kundalini energy. In reality, it is the oldest record of Kundalini yoga. While it is not exactly the Kundalini yoga currently known to mankind, all the foundational elements, pertaining to a Kundalini awakening, are contained within the Vedas. The following will be a yogic interpretation of Vedic teachings, it is not the only understanding of the concepts, principles, and deities from the Vedas, and it is only one of the multi-dimensions of knowledge contained within the Vedas.

Within the Vedas we do find a variety of names and references to the Kundalini, as well as to various related serpent energies that constitute one of the main groups of

Vedic deities; while these are too numerous to list; an example would be *Shaya*[1] in the Rig Veda. But the most important Vedic deity associated with the Kundalini is Agni and Surya. Agni or the inner fire and power of speech and mantra can refer directly to the Kundalini energy (which is also the power of mantra), while Surya is not the Kundalini per se; it is the Kundalini in its triumph or full awakening, having reached the *sahasrara chakra*. Surya is the Kundalini having moved to the crown chakra. This is often referenced as the sun being hidden and revealed in the Vedic journey.

Within numerous later yoga texts, we find references to the Kundalini/Surya connection. Within the *Hatha Yoga Pradipka*, the Kundalini is often described as having the brilliance of a thousand suns. While some systems place more importance on the heart than the crown chakra, this is not in conflict. In reality, the heart and crown chakra are connected via a nadi known as *chitta nadi*. This explains the strong association of the sun (Surya) with the head (crown chakra) and the heart (anahata chakra). We find teachings of the sacred Mount Meru within Hinduism. From a yogic perspective, the sacred Meru is represented physically by the spinal column. In a variety of ancient texts Meru is given a specific height, and located within an ocean, surrounded by seven islands. The seven islands are the seven primary chakras, and Meru is the spinal column or the *Sushumna* of the astral body. Within the *Shiva Samhita,* the sun is referred to as being at the bottom of Meru (II.10), which is the location of the Kundalini energy.

The journey of awakening the Kundalini begins with Ushas. Ushas represents the dawn or more correctly the spiritual dawn. She is our aspiration toward spiritual awakening. The spiritual journey begins with the grace of the spiritual dawn. Though she is called a variety of names in different cultures, in all systems of truth, Ushas is the aspiration for realization.

---

[1] Shayu is a reference to a snake, in particular a boa, and shaya is a reference to sleeping.

Once our aspiration is strong enough, we begin one of the great Vedic battles: The battle between Indra and Vrtra. The Vedic battle between Indra and Vrtra is our internal battle between our higher spiritual desires and the ego. Indra is the warrior (our higher consciousness) that defeats Vrtra (who is the brother or shadow of Indra — ego); the victory of Indra releases the waters. This is one of the main Vedic stories of slaying a dragon (destroying the veiling powers or avarana shakti), and releasing the seven rivers to flow into the sea. The releasing of the waters is the release of knowledge. Vrtra also represents the Kundalini when it is asleep, and its energy is blocked. Indra represents the awakening and release of that energy.

The battle between Indra and Vrtra opens the way for several additional Vedic deities, which are namely Vayu and the Ashvins. Vayu is the deity of the air, which indicates that it is the ruler of prana, the life-force energy. Within the Rig Veda it is taught that the Ashvins are responsible for the movement of the sun (Surya — soul). They are responsible for the movement of Agni to the state or transformation into the state of Surya. The awakening of the Kundalini involves the prana, not just prana itself, but specific forms of prana, called prana and apana in yoga, which are represented by the Ashvins. The Ashvins represent healing, which is one of the qualities of theses two major forms of prana. It is the two major forms of prana (Ashvins) that is responsible for the Kundalini awakening; and their ruler is Vayu, the lord of prana.

As mentioned earlier, Indra's victory over Vrtra releases the waters, the Ashvins connection or pranic connection is indicated within the Rig Veda 1.116.22, which refers to the Ashvins as raising the water from the bottom of the well. This is a direct reference to the raising of the Kundalini. Indra releases the seven rivers, which are the nadis or channels of the seven chakras.

Another Vedic deity of great importance for the Kundalini awakening is Soma. The meaning of Soma is quite varied, and ranges in meaning from plant essence to astral nectars. As was mentioned earlier, Agni is the Kundalini, but Agni is also the first deity to be invoked to drink of Soma. From a yogic/astral perspective, Soma drips down the Sushumna (spinal column) and is consumed in the manipura chakra (3rd chakra). From a yogic standpoint, pertaining to Kundalini awakening, this process is stopped, and the Soma is retained in the higher chakras namely the Sahasrara and the Ajna (6th & 7th). The practice of yoga is the pressing of the soma, and the Kundalini awakening is the drinking of soma from a subtle astral perspective. While Vedic yoga does not address Kundalini yoga per se; it does so in a variety of different forms, as previously discussed. Additionally, Vedic yoga clearly uses pranayama, mantra, and mediation; for some students, there are three questions that might come to mind: 1) Did the Vedic teachings contain yogic techniques that have become lost over the millennia? 2) Was the physical a part of the system, but preserved orally through other traditions? 3) Or was the Vedic form of yoga from the last world age, and did not require the initial preparatory techniques that would become critical in our current age? The current evidence points to probably all three. Clearly, there is evidence that techniques such as mantra, pranayama, and meditation were the essence of the Vedic culture. In fact, the entire Sanskrit alphabet can be practiced using various techniques to awaken the Kundalini energy.

Looking at recent archaeological evidence, we see postures such as sitting crossed legged (*siddhasana* posture, which is very important to present day yoga) present on various seals from ancient India. It is not difficult to speculate that the other postures would have been persevered by other systems just as systems such as Vedic Astrology and Ayurveda are preserved by the different Vedangas and Upavedas[2] today. Again, as the

---

[2] Vedangas are limbs of the Vedas and Upavedas are secondary Vedas such as Ayurveda.

Vedas are a mantric teaching, it cannot be expected to carry specific information on particular techniques, but the broader tradition preserved this information, and the broader tradition eventually evolved into what initially appears to be a separate system. But in reality, it is an extension of the Vedas; as the Vedas are the spiritual authority for Hinduism. In addition, we know that several Vedic seer families have a yogic connection such as Kashyap, Vamadeva, Vashishta and others. In fact, the lineages of all ancient Yoga traditions are entirely Vedic with Hiranyagarbha, Vasistha, Shakti, Krishna and other Vedic figures being the basis of Patanjali and other yogic lines.

The most compelling evidence comes from the *Bhagavad Gita* itself. Within the Gita (4.1) Krishna states "...Imam vivasvate yogaṁ proktavān aham avyayam, vivasvān manave prātha manur ikṣvā kave bravīt." Krisha states, loosely translated, "I have spoken this yoga to Vivasvat, Vivasvat passed [communicated] it to Manu, Manu related it to Ikshvaku..." Here we see a clear reference to yoga's connection to the Vedic lineage, and yogic information being passed downward through the traditional Vedic lineage. This is a compelling statement that a form of yoga was present within the oldest Vedic traditions. While Krishna is the great teacher of Yoga, Patanjali is presented only as a compiler of older yogic teachings.

In reality, modern day Kundalini yoga is just another form of the Vedic Yajna or ritual. It contains internal and external elements, though not the physical fire of the Vedic ritual, it relies on a more internal manifestation of fire and favors more internal approaches achieved through outward techniques such as asana. Kundalini yoga within modern society is an expression of the first words of the Rig Veda 1.1.1, "AUM Agnim īle..." which means, "I worship Agni."[3]

Endnotes for Ushas

Rg Veda 1.92.1

(1) Frawley, David, "The Flow of Soma", www.vedanet.com/Soma.htm

All translations and transliterations are by Yogi Baba Prem unless otherwise noted.

Svara Yoga

Svara is another yoga system not well known to modern society. It primarily focuses on the breath, breath cycle and assigns qualities, attributes, and proper actions with the breath. One of the main texts of Swara Yoga is called the *Shiva Svarodaya.*
In verse 16,

> Svare vedāśca shāstrāṇi svare gāndharvasuttamam.
> Svare ca sarvam trailokyam svarāmātmasvarupakam.

Svara contains the Vedas, Shastras and musical knowledge (and of subtleties).

Svara and the sun, moon, soma juice, are the three worlds. Svara is the soul in form. — *Shiva Svarodaya.*

Clearly we can see a Vedic connection with all of these yoga systems. Though each system is quite different in its view and approach to realization, they do share a common Vedic background.

Different Manifestations of Vedic Yoga

The Mother of other Yoga Systems

Vedic yoga is a more advanced system of yoga. Usually, students move into the practice of Vedic yoga after many years of study and practice with other yoga systems. As an example, Hatha and the physical practices of other yoga systems is critical for the purification and strengthening of the body and mind for the practice of Vedic Yoga. So for most students, it is important to have a yoga practice established before beginning this system.

Earlier it was mentioned that Vedic yoga had four common practices:

1. Mantra. (Repetition of sacred sounds)
2. Pranayama. (Control of the breath)
3. Dhyana. (Meditation)
4. Yajna. (Offerings)

From the standpoint of mantra, the repetition of sounds has a purifying and awakening effect on the mind and body. The Rig Veda alone consists of over 10,000 mantras, with other texts containing thousands more. So it would be literally true to say that Vedic yoga has a mantra for every person and situation they would ever encounter in life.

Mantra and Vedic yoga can be used in a variety of situations and needs. It is commonly used in Vedic astrology (Jyotisha) as remedials and as an important tool to balance the planetary energies. Mantras can also be used to try and limit or affect planets malefic effects on a physical, emotional, or spiritual level.

Mantras are commonly used in Ayurveda. They can be used to balance the tri-dosha, to open nadi's, to affect the chakras and to increase/decrease or balance elements. There are several mantras that are commonly used as powerful healing mantras. These are best learned from a qualified Vedic teacher or Vedic counselor, as they require proper pronunciation.

Each mantra has a particular breathing rhythm that is performed while chanting the mantra. While this is not as common a factor with shorter mantras, it does still pertain to them, and it is critical for chanting longer mantras. So each repetition of a mantra is a pranayama or an exercise in breath control.

Dhyana or meditation is an important technique within this system. It can involve many different approaches; such as the visualization of a particular deity (more will be covered on the concept and purpose of deities later.) It can include the visualization of various symbols that convey important messages to the subconscious mind. A common practice in yoga is called *Trataka*, or gazing. Commonly, this is performed with a ghee flame or candle. This common yogic exercise is a later manifestation of the Vedic Agni and fire ceremonies. But within the Vedic yoga system it would commonly be performed with an image of a deity or deity symbol such as fire.

Yajna has little exposure in our society; as a relatively small number of students are exposed to it, but yet it is one of the most important teachings within this system of yoga. Yajna literally means to worship, or praise, an act of devotion. Commonly, the word sacrifice is used; this has little relevance to western students, but is important in terms of the inner offerings (*Antar yajna*).

Yajna's consists of two primary forms of offerings:

Antar Yajna is the inner offering to divine consciousness.
Bahir Yajna is the outer offering to divine consciousness.

Let's begin with an exploration of the outer offering (Bahir

Yajna). For this purpose a Vedic ceremony called "Agnihotra" will be used. This is a common Vedic fire ceremony, usually performed in the morning and evening at sunrise and sunset.

Analysis of the Vedic ceremony called Agnihotra

Agnihotra is one of the most ancient of Vedic ceremonies, appearing with lengthy commentaries within the Brahmanas. It means the method of invocation (hotra) for Agni, or the sacred fire. While Agnihotra is not as commonly practiced today and is relatively unknown to modern society, the basic concept and methodology continues to manifest within Ayurveda and yoga practices in modern society under different names.

History

Ancient Vedic texts called the Brahmanas present Agnihotra not as a set ceremony, but offer a variety of different ceremonies as Agnihotra. These different ceremonies differ in form and function producing different results for the practitioner. Such forms of Agnihotra are also hinted at the in the Rig Veda. Ancient Agnihotras could be daily, monthly, seasonally, yearly or even many yearlong rituals as indicated in the Brahmanas. This indicates a sophisticated understanding and presentation for the ancient practitioner, where each variation served a particular form and function compared with our modern statistical average "one form fits all" mentality.

While many of the Brahmanas present Agnihotra as an outer form or ritual, it is important to note that all these works can be interpreted from an inner perspective; requiring no ritualistic skill. Some Agnihotras were performed outwardly with the use of various offerings. Others were inner rituals or yoga practices using offerings of speech (mantra), breath (pranayama) or mind (meditation). In reality, the inner ritual or form is considered more advanced and powerful. Both forms were offered to meet the mentality of the practitioner, who might perform any number of these.

Such Agnihotra rituals and the Brahmana texts may provide the basis for later Tantric philosophy as well, which uses their forms and terminology. The term *Svaha* commonly used in tantra is actually the feminine side or consort of Agni, as discussed earlier. The male/female polarity so common within the Tantric system also pervades the Vedic system. This includes not only the Goddesses or feminine sides of the Gods, but dual powers like Agni and Soma, Mitra and Varuna, or the Ashvin twins that comprehend all dualities. In fact, Vedic mantras and the mysticism of the Sanskrit language (the Vedic language) is more prominent in Tantra than in other later Yoga schools. There is additional evidence of Tantric roots within the Vedic teachings. It is possible that the Tantric system merely contains information that was not preserved in the Vedic samhitas or Brahmanas, which allude to many other teachings and hidden meanings. This is an important consideration to counter the tendency of western scholars, few of them practitioners, to separate the different Vedic components from the actual practice of the teachings. In reality, the different systems of Hinduism should not be separated, but are more correctly facets of the same jewel.

Modern day Agnihotra

Modern day Agnihotra is experiencing a revival of the ritualistic form of the practice, done on a daily basis. While rituals still remain foreign to the masses of modern society, numerous movements have started to introduce rituals to increasing numbers of eastern and westerners practitioners. Agnihotra is starting to make in roads with the masses, though it still has a considerable distance to travel before being accepted in modern society.

Modern practitioners are starting to see and appreciate the logic of the Agnihotra ritual, and many are starting to appreciate the purification that comes from the practice of Agnihotra even at an outer level. From a Vedic view, this action is critical in purifying the heart and preparing one for higher spiritual awareness and consciousness. This view is accepted in numerous Vedic books and teachings including the Upanishads.

While the modern day form experienced in the west is a simpler and easier form than the lengthier Brahmanic forms, its effectiveness is being professed around the world. The modern version follows the traditional times of sunrise and sunset and suggests two mantras for each time period. This format is a simple, but yet effective presentation and introduction to the traditional Agnihotra. It is important to learn the mantras from someone familiar in Sanskrit, as pronunciation is important in this type of ritual.

Many modern day practitioners are introduced to these programs via homa, which is a fire ceremony. Homas can be performed for a variety of reasons and can be used in

- Ayurveda
- Vastu
- Jyotish (Vedic Astrology)
- Health
- Business Success
- Marriage
- Spiritual growth (This being the most important.)

In addition, homas can be performed for all the Vedic and Hindu deities, as-well-as achieving particular goals in life.

Inner Form and Ayurveda

While much of the research that has been performed has been on the external form of Agnihotra, it is important to note that there is an internal (antar) form of Agnihotra. The inner form can appear as a meditative form of the outer ritual. A mixture of the inner and outer form appears in Ayurveda, as the strengthening of *jatharagni* (the digestive fire). In fact, Ayurveda has a strong emphasis on the physical fire or jatharagni. Without the fire of jatharagni burning bright, aside from physical digestive problems and ama (toxins) accumulation; the mind will begin to become dull and weaken, eventually, resulting in weakened prana, tejas, and ojas on the physical and mental levels.

The inner form of yajna commonly appears within the Upanishads, especially the *Chandogya Upanishad*, as the Upanishads often represent the inner form of the Vedic ritual. But it is within the yoga system that we witness a powerful system of inner and outer Agnihotra presented in a variety of forms. This can manifest as simple breathing exercises or mantras consciously practiced as a form of agnihotra; to the awakening of the kundalini as one of the ultimate forms of agnihotra.

Most modern practitioners of yoga are not even aware that they are practicing a form of agnihotra, or are even aware of its potential for healing and expansion of spiritual awareness. Hopefully with time and nurturing, this will change into a deeper awareness of the spiritual process that is yoga, and yoga will become the agnihotra and homa it was intended to become.[1]

Vedic Fire Ceremonies

There are numerous Vedic ceremonies that vary in length and complexity. These can range in length from minutes to days, weeks, or months to complete. Obviously, the longer

---

[1]**How to get started.**

The process is quite easy, local Hindu mandirs will often offer agni hotras or homas throughout the year. There are several organizations that perform this task in India and then send the ashes to you once the homa has been completed. They can easily be researched on the Internet.

For those that wish to learn how to perform Agnihotra or homas, these are best learned from qualified teachers or Vedic teachers. You can contact Agnihotra.org for information. You can also contact the American Institute of Vedic Studies at vedicinst@aol.com. Universal Yoga and Yogi Baba Prem provides homas and instruction on the proper performance of personal homas. Contact them at universalyoga@cfl.rr.com

An easy way to practice inner yajna is with the CD "Meditations on the Sacred Fire" by Dr David Frawley (Pandit Vamadeva Shastri) and Yogi Baba Prem. This provides an introduction to inner offerings in an easy format using visualization.

programs are not practical for the average student; as they have limited time and resources for the performance of the outer yajna.

Antar Yajna

Inner (Antar) Yajna involves the same principles such as:

1. Mantra. (Repetition of sacred sounds)
2. Pranayama. (Control of the breath)
3. Dhyana. (Meditation)
4. Yajna. (Offerings)

But these are performed on an inner level with virtually no external form or tools, except for possibly the breath, which in a sense is coming from outside the body. This program is quite simple and is almost a self-initiation into Vedic Yoga. If you have difficulty with the mantras, consult with a qualified Vedic teacher or Vedic counselor. Before beginning this practice, fully read and complete the book at least once.

Technique

Visualize the dawn and hold that image in your mind while chanting:

Om uṣase namaḥ

Then visualize the sun continuing up a little further into the sky and chant the Gayatri mantra:

Om bhur bhuvaḥ svaḥ
tat saviturvareṇyam
bhargo devasya dhīmahi
dhiyo yo naḥ pracodayāt

Then visualize a flame coming out of the sun and into your heart center, as you chant:

Om raṁ agnaye namaḥ

It is an easy processes for anyone to get started on this journey, as you must have already have been spiritually awakened in-order to pick up this book to begin with. Below is a basic self-starter program into Vedic Yoga. This program will take a minimum of 160 days to complete. The times (number of days) given are minimums. The numbers of repetitions are the maximum number. Most students will need to start with a smaller number of repetitions.

1. Start with mantra to Ushas for a minimum of 40 days. 108 repetitions.
2. Gayatri mantra for a minimum of 40 days. 108 repetitions.
3. Agni mantra for a minimum of 40 days. 108 repetitions.
4. Then combine all three for 40 days. 108 repetitions each.

Again it is important to practice this under the guidance of qualified Vedic teacher, as pronunciation is very important, it is critical to learn the proper pronunciation.

Technique Review

Mantra to Ushas

Om uṣase namaḥ

Gayatri Mantra.

Om bhur bhuvaḥ svaḥ
tat saviturvareṇyam
bhargo devasya dhīmahi
dhiyo yo naḥ pracodayāt

The gayatri mantra is available on our "Navagrah-nine planets" CD, available from Universal Yoga. There are also numerous tapes and CD's that contain the mantra available from stores.

Mantra to Agni.

Om raṁ agnaye namaḥ

After successfully completing each mantra for 40 days, then they can be combined into a full program:

Complete Program: Start after 160 days minimum of the previous programs. Do not practice more than 108 repetitions of each mantra.

Om uṣase namaḥ. (maximum 108 repetitions.)

Om bhur bhuvaḥ svaḥ
tat saviturvareṇyam
bhargo devasya dhīmahi
dhiyo yo naḥ pracodayāt. (maximum 108 repetitions.)

Om raṁ agnaye namaḥ. (maximum 108 repetitions.)

Deities

Deity is often a difficult term for modern society. The current mentality, of some people, seems to be in conflict with association with deities. Regrettably, the majority of people do not understand what the term deity is conveying. The term is actually *deva*. Deva literally means heavenly, to shine, worthy of worship, a divine man, or a title among other definitions. In reality, deva does not translate well into English, which is a problem with so many Sanskrit words. A careful examination of deities and their true meaning will reveal their relevance, form, and function within every person's life. As manifestations of Dharma or the highest truth, they transcend religious and cultural dogma manifesting on every level of consciousness.

Within Hinduism the number of deities is quite expansive. Traditionally within Hinduism, the number of deities is 33 million, which is a very high number. Within the Rig Veda, the number of deities is 33, ultimately resulting in four receiving the most focus within the Vedic yoga system. These four are:

1. Indra.
2. Agni.
3. Surya.
4. Soma.

It is important to note that other deities are just as important, or play vital roles in our spiritual, emotional, and physical health. As an example, deities such as Varuna, Ushas, Rudra, and Aditi are very important. To illustrate this point, before we explore the major Vedic deities, let's examine one deity named Ushas and then Varuna.

The Glory of Ushas

To the modern reader, the Hindu pantheon can be a daunting subject to approach. Numerous books have been written on Hindu deities. Many of these books often present what appears to be conflicting information. These conflicts and misunderstandings can even appear within the Eastern mind. There is little wonder that many students give up, frustrated and confused; trying to understand the great teachings of such important works such as the Vedas and others. The key is simply taking the time to understand the symbolic language of ancient teachings and the inner and outer teachings they contain. With the right application of knowledge, the Hindu deities will have a practical and purposeful place within the hearts of all students. The most fundamental place to start with in the understanding of Vedic deities is with Ushas, the spiritual dawn.

Before we can begin to understand an issue as complex as the Vedic deities and their importance, some background information is necessary. The Western scholar has been tremendously influenced by commentaries by Sayana and Yaska. While this is not initially a problem, western scholars have taken their works as the final words on these ancient texts, and this is where the problem begins. Sayana and Yaska both offer commentaries from the viewpoint of a naturalistic religion. In other words, everything they are referencing is a literal or natural phenomenon. There is nothing wrong or incorrect in offering a naturalistic view toward the Vedas; however, it is important to note this was not the only view. In fact, both Sayana and Yaska refer to other commentaries or views existing. To begin to understanding the Vedic mindset, we must realize that they were "Animist", in other words, they saw divinity everywhere. This leads to an inner and outer manifestation of divinity. The inner and outer manifestation of divinity is a fundamental principle of the Vedic teachings. The naturalistic presentation of Sayana and Yaska was a commentary on the Vedic ritual, which initially is an outward expression. But, it is important for the student of the Vedic teachings to develop an appreciation of the outer and inner application of the teachings. To begin this process let us start with a basic understanding to the outer and inner aspects of one deity, Ushas.

The Outer Meaning of Ushas

Ushas is often an overlooked Vedic deity. She is one of the representations of the Goddess in the Vedic system. Though critics often state that there is no feminine representation in the Vedas, this is clearly not true. Ushas, in the Vedas was the dawn. This period of time was considered auspicious for rituals, and especially for yoga and meditative practice. The period approximately two hours before sunrise is called the 'Wind of Brahman" in the yogic system. This is a reference to more prana being available, among other things. After completing important spiritual practices in the pre-dawn hours, Ushas indicated a physical manifestation of an inward process. The dawn represented the growing or increasing light within the practitioner. So even in the outer meaning, Ushas was still very important.

She represents the beginning of light for the day, as the sunrise marked the beginning of the Vedic day. All astrological calculations pertaining to which lunar day was in effect were based on the sunrise times. Her importance is clearly illustrated by her association with light. Light is an important spiritual principle in almost all the worlds' major religions. Ushas representing the beginning of light, the dawn, and sunrise is an important spiritual principle that has its place of prominence within the Vedic ritual and spirituality as a whole.

Inner Meaning of Ushas

The root to Ushas comes from the word *vas*. Vas literally means to shine. With the root meaning to shine and the importance of the Sun in ancient teachings, it is easy to see why Ushas is an important principle and goddess. While the dawn marks the period of time when the day begins, the word shine can mean more on an inner level.

Ushas being the dawn represents our dawning or spiritual awakening. It marks the beginning of a greater inner journey of spiritual realization. We may experience Ushas on a variety of levels. In other words, one may experience the dawn (awakening to things), numerous times in their life. So Ushas is not just the beginning of one journey, she marks the beginning of a variety of journey's and steps on the spiritual path. With this understanding of Ushas, we see that she appears in all spiritual traditions under various names and forms. In fact, we all experience Ushas on a regular basis; as she is present whenever we awaken to a fact or knowledge. Ushas also represents our awakening to the reality of our true nature. She can also represent a form of divine inspiration, though this is more commonly associated with Sarasvati; it would be more correct to recognize Ushas as our aspiration. She can also represent illumination. Ushas represents the end of the night. Night is a metaphor for ignorance (*avidya*), or is commonly interpreted as such. But night can also indicate a period of rest. Ushas, in that case, would make an end to a rest period, and the beginning of a spiritual growth cycle. Likewise, she can also represent our awakening to divine inspiration (Sarasvati).

Ushas can also represent our inner awakening to our purpose in life. The spiritual dawn can represent our awakening to spiritual practices from past lives. This is an essential component for true spiritual awakening. But care is required when awakening to past life spiritual practices, as we have lived in a variety of societies and cultures. Often students awakening to the spiritual path will be drawn to a combination of spiritual paths. This can cause confusion between teachings and the spiritual path.

On a higher level, the spiritual dawn is not a momentary event, or a daily event. In reality, it becomes a conscious state that never disappears. In other words, the dawn becomes continuous. She is the light of truth, or more correctly our recognition of the light of truth and truth itself manifesting in our life.

If one adds Sri Aurobindo's comments on Primitive roots, it is discovered that the primitive root to *vas* is *va*. "Va" literally means "Powerful or Strong". Ushas is not just the beginning of our realization of light; it is also a reminder that this light (truth) is powerful and strong. She is not the weak feminine force in a patriarchal system, but is Shakti itself manifesting throughout the cosmos.

The spiritual dawn is fundamental to human existence, purpose and obtaining the goal of *moksha* (liberation). Each person has within them the aspiration to know the truth. Often there is conflict over the aspiration to know the truth and the ego motivation to control everything. Initially, Ushas is the awakening to our personal desire to seek out the truth. It eventually evolves into a constant state of truth. It is auspicious to invoke the light of dawn, as we begin the path each day.

Observation and Techniques for Understanding Ushas

Almost every person has taken time to appreciate the inner and outer manifestation of Ushas at one time or another; though often they do not know her by name. Though millions of people are driving to work each day at sunrise or shortly after sunrise, few take the time to observe the sunrise or appreciate the dawn hours. But each year we spend large amounts of money on vacation to visit exotic places. It is often during this time that we take the time and appreciate the pre-sunrise and sunrise hours. Somehow it is special with us being away from home. This is a momentary manifestation of the outer appreciation of Ushas. Likewise, few people have taken the time to appreciate the beginning of a journey, especially his or her spiritual journey. Though recognizing the beginning of the spiritual journey is often seen when reflecting back on past events. Even then, in reflection on the past, often people will show a deep sense of appreciation for the beginning of the journey. Almost everyone has had a moment that they felt a strong spiritual realization that provided insight into a problem or guidance. Ushas was the vehicle for the realization.

To accelerate our awakening to deeper levels of divinity, it would be beneficial to perform mantra and visualization to Ushas. The Rig Vedas offers numerous mantras to Ushas. Mantra to Ushas can be best learned from teachers knowledgeable in Sanskrit and the Vedas. In addition, visualization of the dawn can be beneficial. This is an easy and practical technique that can be practiced by almost anyone. The next time one is up early in the morning, take time to think about Ushas and the dawn, reflect on the true meaning and feel that connection with the awakening of divine illumination within yourself.

Ushas has many more attributes and we will examine a few of them here. Literally, a separate book could and should be written on her. It is important to remember, without the coming of the dawn (spiritual awareness) there can be no release from the illusions of the night (ignorance). Ushas marks our personal movement from night into the light of day.

Working with the energy of Ushas is quite simple:

- It can be as easy as chanting to Ushas in the early morning hours.
- Enjoying the sunrise and contemplating the inner meaning of the sunrise and Ushas.
- Meditation visualization of the sunrise, while contemplating Ushas.
- Chanting to Ushas during the auspicious time of just

before sunrise or other time of day. This can also be performed when a person first wakes up, regardless of the time.

- Special chanting of mantras to Ushas during the winter solstice. (Mantras to Ushas should be learned directly from a teacher due to complexity of the Sanskrit language).
- Past Life regression can also be an aid, provided it is practiced in the proper area and for proper purpose.
- Visualization involving a sense of your own personal awakening.
- Visualization of the growing light within the self. Possibly adding a feeling of expansion of this light.
- Affirming the principle of Ushas when you have a revelation or realization about anything.
- Cultivating a desire for spiritual growth through study of ancient texts and with qualified teachers.
- The practice of Yoga and Meditation cultivates our relationship with Ushas.

A Closer Examination of Ushas

Om uṣase namaḥ!!! Each morning when I wake up this mantric thought enters my mind. My awakening is to greet the spiritual dawn. As the day progresses, the spiritual dawn continues. Even in night, the dawn continues to illuminate the path of self-realization. While the physical dawn is but a fleeting moment in time, a snapshot, already in the past by the time that we physically see it. The inner dawn is eternal, ever present, within the hearts of each of us.

The goal becomes to capture the essence of the spiritual dawn (Ushas) and continue to dwell there, to not let the spiritual dawn cease to exist. To consciously remain with the spiritual dawn (truth) at all times.

In the previous chapter, a basic introduction of Ushas was provided. Can there be more to Ushas? Is there more that can be understood from the name Ushas? The answer is yes.

Previously, we explored that the verbal root to Ushas was *vas*, which can mean to shine. It is important to note that *vas* can also mean to dwell, to live or reside in. Again, following Sri Aurobindo's commentaries on primitive roots, the root to *vas* would be *va*. Va literally means powerful or strong. Combining these three concepts together provides powerful insight into Ushas. The three attributes to Ushas are:

1. To Shine
2. To Dwell
3. To be Powerful or Strong.

Adding these three together can provide powerful insight into the deeper meaning of a word. I would propose that a complete relationship with Ushas is to obtain our strength by dwelling within the light, spiritual realization, or learning to dwell in the strong light of consciousness.

A closer examination will reveal that most of the Eastern systems have some slant toward this truth. Ushas is the awakening to the shining truth of reality. Our goal and relationship with Ushas is that the spiritual dawn represents our developing ability to dwell in this powerful state of realization.

Ushas and Agni

Ushas and Agni have an important and powerful relationship. Agni is one of, if not, the most important deities within the Rig Veda. The first mantra within the Vedas is for Agni. Agni can manifest on many levels. On an outer level, the sunrise and fire of the sun would be Agni. The deity that opens the door for this vision is Ushas. The dawn prepares the world for the arrival of light. The dawn (Ushas) is our aspiration to see the light, and the perception and digestion of light is Agni. Ushas is the preparation for the Vedic fire ceremony, and the actual fire is Agni. Agni manifests within the three worlds, and its highest state is the Sun or soul. Again our aspiration for this state is nurtured by Ushas.

In the Rig Veda 1.48.15 there is a reference to Ushas opening the doors to *divah*, which means opening the doorway to *dyau* or the heavens, light, or fire. This is a clear reference to Ushas opening our awareness to the subtle body. While the word *dvar* means a door or gate, it also means the way or access. Again, we see a hidden relationship between Agni, the fire, and Ushas opening the doors to higher levels of consciousness.

Ushas and the relationship with the Kundalini

Ushas, while not being the Kundalini, is directly associated with the Kundalini energy. There are teachings that the Kundalini is responsible for all realizations that we have. In teaching, I have often ıeferred to this as the Kundalini "pulsing", but not a true awakening of the Kundalini energy. The difference between "pulsing" and the awakened Kundalini has led to much confusion in modern society about the Kundalini. Often, a teacher will comment on a student having a vision, a realization, and will state it was the Kundalini. This is not to imply that the student has had a full Kundalini awakening, but that the energy was released in a tiny proportion. The "pulsing' is a very small release of energy that travels up the sushumna (spine), or just barely into the sushumna. The physical/mental manifestation of this is the experience of the "light bulb" going off in our head.

Ushas more correctly represents the awakening of the Kundalini, and ultimately the ability to stay in the awakened state. The practice of Kundalini yoga is a system using different terminology to cultivate Ushas awakening in our life. Again, we see the important relationship between Ushas and Agni. As Agni, in the Vedas, is the Kundalini, as well.

Ushas and the Chakras

Ushas as a lower physical manifestation would be associated with the manipura chakra (3rd) i.e. sight. Ushas as a higher physical manifestation would manifest with the Ajna chakra (6th) spiritual sight. This also emphasizes the relationship with Agni and Ushas again, as Agni is responsible for the digestion of light. These include the different levels of sight and perception. It would be associated with desire; in the case of Ushas, it is the desire for truth. If we look at Ushas from the *Samkhya*[1] system, Ushas would be associated with the Tanmatras. In addition, all the yogic techniques for awakening the higher function of Buddhi would all have Ushas leading the process. Ushas would manifest in the anahat chakra (4th) as the quality of higher love, and devotion, the aspiration to realize the true nature of the self.

---

[1]Samkhya is one of the 6 major systems that comprise Hinduism.

This view takes us into the multidimensional aspects of Vedic deities. The Vedic deities can represent abstract spiritual truths, principles and form. Likewise, they can manifest on a multitude of different attributes, aspects, and forms. As the Vedic deities represent universal truth (Dharma), their manifestation can be found in a multitude of forms. That is one function of the 108 or 1008 names of deities. The numerous names represent the manifestation of the deity and its attributes on a variety of levels. This allows for a shishya (student) to have an *Ishtadevata* (an *ishtadevata* is the personal deity that one may choose to follow). As an example, if we view Shiva as only the destroyer, then one would only go to Shiva for issues relating to destruction, and even many people's views towards Shiva as the destroyer can be quite limited; not encompassing the rich teachings regarding the purpose of the destroyer. Shiva represents much more than this one concept or idea. Shiva can represent peace, among many other things also. The numerous names introduce the student or devotee to the numerous other attributes and functions of the one deity.

Ushas and the Vedas

There are numerous hymns to Ushas within the Rig Veda. While the number of suktas (hymns) cannot be a correct reflection of importance, clearly the importance of Ushas cannot be added or subtracted due to the number of hymns.

Ushas is associated with the middle world (*antariksh* — atmosphere), and she is also strongly associated with pranic level of the body (Rig Veda 1.92.1). In one part of the Rig Veda (1.92.1), it was mentioned that there were several dawns within ones life. This verse deals specifically with that issue. The word *ushasah* is used implying a plural sense: dawns. It is not just a dawn, but many dawns. This verse implies that the sages had experienced many stages of higher consciousness. This is very important, as the spiritual path and path towards realization does often consist of many moments of spiritual awakening.

Ushas is also referenced with Soma in the Rig Veda (1.49.1). This sukta references Usha coming from dyau (the heavenly plane) to the home of soma (...tvā somino grham — you to the home of soma). The home of Soma occurs on several levels, the astral body being one important home from a spiritual standpoint. It is the flow of soma that sustains the body, the restriction of the flow of soma from its downward flow to the third chakra, in yogic teachings, truly nourishes the body, as well as the mind. Physically, the soma would be the nectar within the brain and Ushas arrival would be conscious realization. This is illustrated by Pandit Vamadeva Shastri (Dr. David Frawley), "Soma, according to the Vedas, flows in a thousand streams" (1). This would involve Agni as well, but it is Ushas that opens the door for the relationship between Agni and Soma. Whereas Soma is the deity behind Ojas (vitality) and Bhakti (devotion), it is Ushas that is the doorway to Bhakti. Bhakti increases Ojas within the physical body, and the key to this is Ushas, our love, peace and aspiration for divinity.

Ushas in Vedic Astrology

Ushas is the consort of the Sun, or Surya. She has her place within the realm of Vedic astrology. While her role is not as apparent to many, and little interest is currently given to her. Everyone desires her blessings. In reality, she is the higher form of Kama (desire), in the form of aspiration. It would be good to invoke her just as Brihaspata (Jupiter) is invoked at the beginning of an astrological remedial or Puja.

Her relationship with the Sun indicates her ability to open the doorways to self-realization of the soul (Atman/Purusha). The higher function of the Sun is soul awareness, or cosmic awareness. She also assists on the lower level of the sun, which is ego; Ushas and her awakening quality, aids to transform the lower sun (ego) into an awareness of the higher sun (atman). It is Ushas silently working in the subconscious mind that brings the aspirant to their personal experience of oneness with the Sun.

Conclusion

Ushas is an important Vedic deity. While the other Vedic deities represent the process, she marks the aspiration for the other deities. She is strong and powerful. She is one of many that represent the Goddess within the Vedic system. She is the shining light that guides each of us along the path, or at least the beginning awareness of the light. She has an important relationship with primary deities such as Agni and Soma. Without Ushas dwelling within each of us, no one would bring the shining light of realization, aspiration, love and peace to our conscious mind. Ushas is with every deity, silently serving humankind throughout the yugas (world-ages).

An Extended Examination of Ushas

Ushas and the Western World

Hinduism's impact on the United States has been tremendous from a spiritual standpoint. As important teachers such as Vivekananda and Yogananda led the way for many important teachers to travel to United States and teach. This has resulted in the *New-Age* movement to be largely based on and influenced by Hinduism.

If one were to examine the relationship between Ushas and the United States, the importance of the same quickly becomes clear. Let's begin with an examination of the word:

उषस्   Ushas in Sanskrit.

The United States of America is abbreviated as USA. It is also correct to spell in transliteration Ushas — Usha or uìa. The name of Ushas, and the abbreviation of our country is the exact same.

The spiritual dawn should be ruling or influencing power of the United States and reflects this country's spiritual awakening and religious embrace of Hinduism — though often through the form of the New-Age movement. This has lead to spiritual prosperity in the United States (Usa), though clearly it has had its cloudy days and moments.

One of the great attributes that has aided in the manifestation of Ushas within the United States is the "separation of the church and state." While many argue that this concept infringes on religion, in reality it fully protects all religions, minority and large based religions. The separation of church and state allows Ushas to blossom. More importantly, it allows Ushas to blossom within the hearts and minds of society.

In fact, groups that try and infringe on separation of church and state are more oriented toward destruction of Ushas than the expansion of consciousness or spiritual growth of the masses. Every spiritual seeker should promote the preservation of Ushas within the fabric of the United States.

The same process is well underway in Europe. Hinduism and Hindu teachings are experiencing explosive growth. Ushas has inspired many students in Europe to embrace yoga, ayurveda and Vedic astrology. Classes and numerous schools for Vedic teachings are expanding throughout Europe. In reality, Europe has been even quicker than the United States to embrace more esoteric teachings, mysticism, and numerous teachings founded in Hinduism.

Mantras to Ushas

There are numerous suktas (hymns) to Ushas within the Rig Veda, but for the beginner, the best mantra to start with would be:

Om uṣase namaḥ
(Ohm OO-sha-say na-ma-ha)

This mantra can be performed while visualizing the dawn. It can also be chanted during the dawn or pre-dawn hours, as this would be most auspicious. Mantra to Ushas can be practiced during other times of day also, though the dawn and pre-dawn hours are best.

Additional notes on Ushas

While Ushas is the spiritual and literal dawn, she is also the sister of night; indicating her ability to appear during the darkness of night (ignorance) and deliver her light. She has been viewed as the breath of life for the Vedas, indicating her association with prana. The variety of colors in the dawn and pre-dawn sky represent the cosmic rays (cows) held sacred within the Hindu religion (Sanatana Dharma). Some teachings state that cows drive her chariot. The cow is symbolic for knowledge. Again, this illustrates the divine rays (cows) emanating from her; and it is important for us to remember that she is the consort of the Sun. Visually, she is often described as wearing red robes and a golden veil, which illustrates her ability to embrace Rajas (activity) and Sattva (balance) for the student of meditation. She can manifest during the tamasic state especially during times of desperation. As often people have spiritual breakthroughs during challenging times or times that are emotional lows. While Ushas is not associated directly with Tamas, she does manifest as a bridge between the suffering state of tamas and open the doorways to the rajasic state (to make changes in one's life) or the sattvic state, obtaining greater harmony within one's life.

She could be likened to Kali also, but more correctly it would be that she is the sister of Kali. In this case, the dark form of Kali representing the transforming form of Kali from ignorance (transformation from ignorance to realization) that is initialized by the light of Ushas, which eventually brings the aspirant to the lighter form of Kali, which exists in abstract consciousness. This can also be the higher form of the dark Kali. Kali can be explored on much deeper and insightful levels, but that is beyond the scope of this book.

Conclusion

We have examined Ushas in some detail in this book. We have seen her manifestation on an inner and outer level. We have seen her work with the Kundalini, the chakras and touched on her relationship with other deities. Ushas resides within each person; it only takes a small effort to see her. Many have seen her and did not know her name. But all will witness her at one point or another in their spiritual awakening. Next, we will explore the relationship between Ushas and yoga.

Ushas and Yoga

Ushas can manifest within the yoga and Ayurvedic system on every level. Upon careful examination, one will discover that Ushas is an important Vedic deity, and important within the yogic systems. While there is little direct reference to Ushas within yogic texts, it is difficult to believe that she does not exist within the yogic system. Especially, when one considers that Yoga is one of the six *Vedic Darshanas* (six Vedic philosophical systems). In this light, it is difficult to believe that yoga should be something separate from the Vedic teachings, especially when one considers that Vedic yoga is the mother yoga of all other systems. Even the yogic practice of arising before sunrise and practicing yoga is an Ushas ceremony. Ushas does manifest in a variety of different systems and teachings. According to the Rig Veda:

> etā utyā uṣasaḥ ketumakrata pūrve ardhe rajaso bhānumañjate
> These dawns have created light. Rig Veda 1.92.1

What is interesting in this verse is the plural form of dawn, it indicates many dawns of Ushas; implying that in ones spiritual journey, numerous dawns will manifest within their life, not just literal dawns, but spiritual realizations. This is the domain of Ushas. To truly understand Ushas, one must see her manifest on a multitude of levels and degrees of consciousness.

Ushas and the Five Koshas

Within yogic philosophy exists five koshas or sheaths.

These sheaths form the components of the physical, astral, and causal body. An extensive philosophical system is built around these sheaths, and they are well worth additional study. The five koshas are:

1. Annamaya kosha
2. Pranamaya kosha
3. Manomaya kosha
4. Vijnanamaya kosha
5. Anandamaya kosha

Annamaya Kosha

Anna means food, so Annamaya kosha is the food sheath. Ushas manifests knowledge on a lower level with recognizing the need to exercise and take care of the body, as well as the body being the vehicle of consciousness in the physical world. A modern example of this is the fitness craze that currently exists in modern society. This phase is not rooted in a search for health or to maintain the physical body, but is more an obsession with appearance. The obsession over physical appearance is a derangement of the Annamaya kosha. Over time or incarnations, this evolves into the intermediate and higher manifestations of Ushas. This manifests with the desire to eat healthy, exercise in order to maintain health and wellness without cosmetic considerations. Then Ushas and awakening eventually evolves into a vegetarian diet and an incorporation of more sattvic (harmonious) qualities. The body becomes viewed as a temporary temple for the soul. It is given foods and nourishment from a spiritual standpoint, and to increase prana within the body. At this point, Ushas is beginning to cross over into the second sheath, Pranamaya kosha.

Pranamaya Kosha

Pranamaya kosha is the pranic sheath of the body. It is the body's energy and vitality. Just as the foods and consumption of liquids determines the amount of prana the body can carry.

Ushas in the lower manifestation is awakening knowledge of basic breathing exercises. Usually these are for stress reduction, anxiety, and relaxation.

In higher manifestations Ushas brings realization of pranayama, visualization, meditation, mantra, and control of the mind and senses, especially control of the prana. It is at this point she is crossing over into the third kosha, Manomaya kosha.

Manomaya Kosha

Manomaya kosha is the sensory impressions and lower functions of the mind. As pranayama, meditation and other techniques associated with the previous kosha continue, Ushas manifests as the need to move back and control sensory impressions. As the higher knowledge through Ushas begins to manifest, one may start to desire to move away from negative friends, negative experiences. One may desire more quiet time. Ushas in an even higher level brings a need to be near sacred places, or holy people. Listening to sacred teachings or scriptures becomes more important, and one would recognize that need. This can also manifest as desires for meditation, especially deeper meditative states. This is the manifestation of Ushas on the higher levels. This awakens the desire to develop intellectual knowledge.

Vijnanamaya Kosha

This is the realm of the intellect. The limitations of Manomaya kosha are being reduced and the ability to resolve issues without an emotional action or reaction becomes stronger in this function. Ushas awakens one to the desire to study and understand teachings. She can manifest within the intellect as awakenings as one moves along the path of study. Her lower manifestation is basic beginner spiritual books, teachings and systems. While lower, this is an important step, as we all must begin somewhere in the journey of self-realization.

Anandamaya Kosha

This is the realm of bliss. The lower manifestation is the human orgasm, which is only a momentary glimpse into a spiritual state. Over time, this should inspire one to seek higher states of consciousness using methods that are more effective and longer lasting than the sexual experience. Ushas manifests as glimpses into higher realms of consciousness, or deeper meditative realizations of love and bliss.

Ushas and Kama

Ushas by her very nature should inspire desire. It is the desire for liberation that is critical to transiting human existence. The Sanskrit word for desire is *Kama*; this word has become misaligned with its lower manifestation, which will be explored later. Without Kama's relationship with Ushas, the spiritual path becomes very difficult. It is desire for the spiritual experience that helps many students to remain on the path. It is the initial spiritual experiences for the beginner that inspires and sows the seed of desire for further growth. This can occur through books, meditation, mantra, or spiritual study. Each dawning and realization through Ushas creates a desire for further study, experience, and realization.

Within Ayurveda, it is taught that there are four aims of life.

1. Dharma
2. Artha
3. Kama
4. Moksha

Dharma is the true teachings of spirituality. Artha is material prosperity and recognition. Kama is often taught as desire and Moksha is liberation. Usually, the masses are focused on one or two of the four aims, primarily Artha and Kama in modern society. Within our modern era, Kama is primarily viewed as lust, desire, affection or sensual love. Coming from the root *Kam*, literally meaning love, is often viewed as lower love. But when combined with Ushas, Kama begins to manifest in its higher form of spiritual aspiration. It is this higher manifestation of Kama that is most important.

Often one can become confused with Kama and spiritual teachings due to the perception that there should be no desires. Looking at the Ayurvedic four aims of life, it is revealed that the first three aims should work to support and manifest the fourth aim. Again, this is teaching Kama in its higher manifestation. Ushas (the dawn) stimulates the higher function of Kama, manifesting as desire for spiritual experience.

In Hinduism, Kama is armed with a bow and arrows indicating his later manifestation as Cupid. He is born of Krishna and Rukmini. The gods selected him as a commander of their forces in the war with a demon, indicating the power of desire for victory against lower forces. His wife is Rati, which in its lower form means pleasure, joy, or delight; in its higher manifestation means devotion. This indicates the important role Kama has within Bhakti yoga, the yoga of devotion.

Kama is also considered to be a name for the Supreme Being, Brahman. This further connects the higher aspects of Kama with devotion and divine love. Kama also has a powerful manifestation with the Vedic deity Agni as Kamagni, the fire of love. In its lower manifestation, it is passion; in its higher manifestation, it is a powerful love for the divinity.

Example's of Kama's higher manifestation

While this is not always true, usually the experience of Kama is preceded by Ushas. Here are a few examples of the manifesting desire after a direct experience with Ushas:

- The longing for spiritual study.
- Desiring the company of spiritual people.
- Desire to learn meditation.
- Desire to learn mantra.
- Desire to purify the mind and body.
- Longing to know the truth.
- Longing for communion with Divinity.
- Seeking out of knowledge.

Kama can also manifest within the eight limbs of Yoga, as

compiled in the "Yoga Sutras of Patanjali".

- **Yama and Niyama**. Kama manifests in the first two limbs called Yama and Niyama as desires to conduct one self properly in social and personal activities.
- **Asana**. Kama manifests as a desire to take care of the body. To detox, increase flexibility, and prepare the body for further spiritual awareness, to begin to cleanse the subtle channels of the body.
- **Pranayama**. Kama is the desire to strengthen the vital organs with the life-force energy. It is a longing or desire to further cleanse the subtle channels of the body called *nadi's*.
- **Pratyahara.** This is the desire to pull the out flowing senses inward. It can manifest as desire to withdraw from sensory stimulation such as mass media, or computers.
- **Dharana.** Kama is the desire to develop concentration, as concentration is essential to experience meditation. This is often experienced in its lower form with concentration on work or school. In its higher form it is concentration on spiritual qualities and teachings.
- **Dhyana.** Kama in the lower form is the desire to meditate. In the higher form it is to seek communion with the higher self or Godhead.
- **Samadhi.** This is the complete bliss of communion with the higher self or Godhead.

Within this system, Agni plays an important role. As mentioned earlier, Kamagni is the fire of love. Agni is an essential component to this sacred formula, as Agni represents digestion; we must be able to digest the experiences (*anubhava*) from Ushas, and the experiences that are a result of the desire following the spiritual dawn. Without Agni, these experiences will have no purpose or understanding to us.

Kama even in its lower form of sexual pursuit is preparing the aspirant for higher study, as all sexual longing and desire is actually rooted in desire for the spiritual experience. Even in its most base manifestation, Kama is preparing the ground for higher spiritual truths and it is Ushas that opens the doorway for this higher manifestation of Kama.

While it is common to attach a deities meaning to one or two levels of understanding or to remain within the naturalistic symbology often used for modern interpretation within the Vedas; it is not far reaching to develop a more expansive understanding of the deities, as well. The *Bhagavad Gita* provides insight into the different manifestations of the deities by examining terms such as *adhibutic, adhiyatmic, etc.*(Bhagavad Gita VIII 1-2). These terms can easily be applied to the deities, as an example the adhibutic level of Ushas is the literal dawn. The adhiyatmic manifestation of Ushas is the psychological and emotional awakening to a higher truth — especially higher spiritual truth.

Ushas and the Vedas

Within the naturalistic symbology of the Rig Veda, Ushas, the divine dawn, marks the beginning of the day and more importantly-sunrise (Surya). Surya is the illumination of the soul. Surya always follows Ushas, as Ushas paves the way for the sun to rise. This is certainly true in the physical world, and the material world is but a reflection of the inner spiritual world. Ushas as the beginning of our spiritual awakening marks the beginning of our spiritual illumination, represented by Surya. This in term gives birth to the divine fire, Agni, within our life; which, in term, takes the practitioner back to "Agni Yoga" which is the foundation of all major spiritual principles.

The challenge facing most spiritual aspirants is not just a spiritual experience, but cultivating the ability to retain the spiritual experience. Or more importantly, the ability to hold a specific vibration generated through the spiritual experience.

But the ability to strongly retain the spiritual experience is one of the important functions of the Vedic Agni. But that is the subject of another book. For the purpose of this study, the process is achieved through multiple dawns. Just as the dawn occurs each morning in the physical world; each spiritual dawn must be experienced regularly or reinforced for it to become rooted in our life. This view is supported by the Rig Veda, which says, "*These dawns have created the light...*" Rig Veda 1.92.1 or in the Rig Veda 1.92.10, it states, "*Again, again, she, the ancient Goddess, is born*". The Rig Veda also identifies three functions and three types of people that Ushas will affect. For the lazy person, she begins the proper course. For the person performing offerings, she stimulates wealth on many levels. For the person having limited view, she extends their view. She also directs people down their vocations and desired objects. (Rig Veda 1.113.5-6)

An Exercise

Visualize your body sitting in a comfortable posture with the legs crossed or sitting straight in a chair. Visualize the color of the dawn emitting from the body through the aura. Let the color be vibrant red hues. Practice this visualization for 10-15 minutes daily.

Once this visualization becomes comfortable, a chant can be added.

Suggested chant: Om uṣase namaḥ

Pronounced (Ohm OO-sha-say na-ma-ha)

Ushas and the Gunas

The Sanskrit word *guna* means attribute. These "attributes" serve as a powerful indicator, and formulator of the physical principles of the earth. The concept of guna is one of the more important teachings from India. These attributes provide powerful insight into our spiritual growth, worldly manifestations, and the formation of matter from the subatomic level into more dense levels of matters manifestation. But most importantly they provide a powerful tool to accelerate personal and planetary transformation.

Within the yoga tradition, the focus is on three primary gunas:

1) Sattva
2) Rajas
3) Tamas

Sattva is balance, harmony, peace and similar qualities. Rajas is activity and movement. It is dynamic. Tamas is inertia, non-moving, and sometimes lethargy. Of these three gunas, yoga embraces the cultivation of sattva. Through sattva, one realizes that one may embrace other gunas at times as needed. As an example, if a person were stuck in a rut (tamas) they would need to embrace some form of activity (rajas) to move from their position of immobility.

In relation to the human psyche, Ushas marks the beginning of each transition of the gunas. Within the lokas of each person the three gunas or combinations of the gunas are at work. As an example, within the field of 'manomaya kosha', an individual might be very lethargic, mentally dull, lazy or similar attribute. By the cosmic force of Ushas activating in their life, they realize that they need to "open their mind" or become more active mentally. They may realize that they are negative and need to adopt a more positive attitude. All of these realizations are rooted in Ushas. Ushas would mark the beginning of their journey from a tamasic mental state to a rajasic. This would usually manifest as a "dual guna type" such as a tamasic/rajas or rajas/tamasic mental type. This view is strongly supported within Ayurveda, as it values the teachings regarding gunas as well.

An excellent example of the integration of Ushas and guna could be found in the annamaya kosha (food sheath). Ushas would provide an awakening from tamasic foods, for instance these foods might be alcohol, meat, heavily processed foods, or foods that were devitalized; to more sattvic type foods, such as fresh fruits and vegetables in our diet.

So taking the five koshas and adding the three gunas for each kosha, we realize that there are fifteen states for the five koshas, excluding the dual combinations. Cultivating a strong understanding of the koshas and the gunas provides a powerful tool for spiritual growth and personal wellbeing. Once one has cultivated a solid foundation of the koshas, one can then begin to examine the different qualities at work within oneself.

Practice Exercise

As an exercise, take time and examine the koshas in your life. Once you have become familiar with them and can see most of them at work, then work to see the gunas the forces of inertia, activity, and balance at work in the world of nature. Once this has become comfortable, combine the two exercises. Take time to explore each guna and kosha.

Conclusion

Ushas, the koshas, and their relationship with the gunas are a broad and expansive subject. We have only touched on a few key issues. But with practice, observation, and patience a great deal can be gained from practicing a broader view of the deities. In a sense, becoming inspired to read this book comes from Ushas, though the inspiration from Ushas most likely started long before reading this book; it is an indication of the Ushas force at work within each of our lives.

Ushas is a dynamic cosmic principle in the personal spiritual journey toward consciousness, which is light. We must first invoke the dawn as we awaken from our slumber. Our journey from the night (spiritual unawareness) into the light of day (consciousness) cannot begin without the transition between night and day through the dawn. Ushas brings this great gift to all people throughout the world. But is Ushas associated with other qualities?

The Secret of Ushas

While we have explored Ushas from a variety of angles, one of the lesser known is the Ushas connection with speech. Ushas is a manifestation of the Vedic deity *Vac* or speech. Within the Vedic tradition, speech is believed to hold a special power. On some levels, the entire Rig Veda is a text on speech. Being a samhita, the Rig Veda has a special connection with speech, sound, and the relationship between sound and form.

Within the Tantric tradition, a great importance is placed on speech, as well. It was common within the darker tantric systems to attack a person's speech. The reason for this is quite clear. With speech comes our ability to create. The sounds we enunciate are believed to hold power within them. Each time we speak, we are in essence creating and manifesting a world; a world of mind and thoughts that can influence others and ourselves powerfully. Speech is one of the most powerful tools in yoga and meditation.

It could be argued that Ushas could be the awakening or recognition of the importance of speech, and the power of speech. The ancient texts are clearly telling us more about the importance of speech. On a spiritual level, the experience of Ushas is commonly experienced through speech. This thread is reflected in the majority of Vedic teachings. As previously mentioned, the Rig Veda is entirely comprised of mantra, which has a speech or sound component. The other Vedic texts also contain mantras and rituals that require speech or sound. The Upanishads literally mean to sit and listen. The entire Upanishads are designed for speech and are manifestations of *Vac*, *Ushas*, and *Sarasvati*.

What is most interesting is the root to Ushas, which is *ush,* meaning to shine; also means to burn. This is a reference to the burning power of speech. Certainly, we have all experienced the burning power of harsh speech. Likewise, the burning power of spiritual speech can cut through the illusions of life, and allow us to awaken to the deeper truth hidden within ourselves.

This power of speech manifests on four primary levels:

1. Vaikhari
2. Madhyama
3. Pashyati
4. Para

Vaikhari is the final stage in the process of speech. It is literal sound that is expressed out into the world. Madhyama means "middle". It is a more subtle level of speech, entering the realm of thought. But more importantly, it is the speech of the subtle body or astral body. Pashyati is the speech of the "spiritual eye". It is of the causal body. This is the speech that comes from really seeing the truth. Para means supreme and is the speech of divine consciousness.

Ushas is strongly linked with each of these levels of speech, especially the more subtle ones. And through the spoken and unspoken power of speech, she awakens us to the power of spirituality. The link between Ushas and speech is indicated in the Rig Veda, 1.48.2, which asks Ushas to speak directly to the aspirant. This would be an excellent mantra to perform.

The connection with Ushas and speech is also reflected in *Krishna Yajur Veda Taittirya Samhita* which states that the "[Ushas} yokes the Gayatri, Trishtubh, Jagati, and Anushtubh..." KYJTS 4.3. This section of the KYVTS continues on referring to the five dawns. One of the meanings to this reference is the connection between Ushas and the five sheaths, which was explored earlier.

Practice Exercise

For those that do not speak Sanskrit, merely close eyes and

visualize a dawn. Visualize numerous red rays of light flowing from the horizon. Then affirm and ask, "Ushas speak to me directly."

It is clear that Ushas is an important deity and plays a vital role in spiritual awakening, realization, and growth on all levels of our being. This point can also be illustrated by a quick study of the Vedic deity called Varuna.

Varuna

The Eastern Teachings of Reincarnation and Karma in Relation to the Vedic Deity Varuna

While the concept of reincarnation has appeared in a variety of cultures and teachings, the Hindu teachings appear to contain the greatest wealth of teachings on this subject. The oldest of this knowledge centers on a Vedic deity known as Varuna.

Varuna is a little known deity in the modern age; but in reality, he is one of the most important Vedic deities, and serves as the father to the somewhat better-known Indra from the Vedas. Varuna was often a feared deity among the ancient people, and for one simple reason: Karma.

Varuna as the lord of karma was perceived as great punisher, and often ancient people prayed to be saved from the wrath of Varuna. While it is true that the ancient people prayed to avoid the wrath of Varuna, in reality, they were praying for an alteration of their karma, which is what many people seek even today. But a closer examination will reveal that Varuna is the greatest friend of humanity, and is the force responsible for the manifestation of the human experience.

While Varuna is the world ruler that oversees the manifestation of karma, without the grace of Varuna, there would be no force to trigger incarnation. Without incarnation there can be no relief or resolution of karma. A perfect example is given in the *Krishna Yajur Veda's Taittiriya Samhita (4.2.10.3* vātasya dhrājim varuṇasya nābhīm*)* which states that "[he is] born of the motion of wind from the navel of Varuna." This is indicating that it is the movement of prana and power from Varuna that results in incarnation. From this standpoint, Varuna comes into illumination as to his importance. Mantra to Varuna is for the purpose of balancing or harmonizing karma. The wrathful form of the deity is not experienced unless we refuse to grow. Then the wrathful form of the deities' energy is required to facilitate growth within the individual or society. Varuna is also a deity of dharma, requiring that he represents truth and the spiritual path. Varuna's association with the path of the fathers (pitririyana) indicates his association with the downward flow of energy into manifestation. In other words, divine energy flowing into creation.

This powerful relationship that Varuna has with manifestation of karma is balanced with numerous mantras being to Mitra and Varuna or Indra and Varuna. In the former, Mitra becomes the force that manages the forces of karma and their manifestation in a more manageable way. Indra as the son of Varuna shapes and molds the manifestation of karma for the individual.

Varuna appears in the Atharva Veda (5.24.4) as a protective power, to obtain knowledge. In other words, one cannot obtain knowledge without the help of karmas. Also the same text (7. 83.2-3) refers to Varuna "loosening the bonds" (karma); the *Atharva Veda* provides clear evidence of Varuna's connection with karma. For working with karma, mantra to Varuna is an important tool, especially when karma is becoming a difficult task to bare, mantra to Mitra and Varuna can provide much needed relief.[1]

We are merely scratching the surface of the depth of the great tradition of Hinduism, now to examine the primary four Vedic deities.

Agni. Agni is considered by many to be the most important Vedic deity, if such a title can be given. Agni manifests on many levels of our being. Within our physical body, Agni is the digestive fire called Jatharagni. On the level of the mind, Agni is our will power. It is the ability to digest experience and activities in our life. Agni is a deity of the fire element providing the power of transformation, as Agni does purify the mind and body. Agni is the kundalini energy when active.

An excellent mantra to Agni is:

Om ram agnaye namaḥ.

Soma. Soma is bliss. It is a nurturing energy that vitalizes our mind and body. It is one of the manifestations of love. It provides vitality, stamina, and joy. Soma is the nectar or amrit of the yoga systems. It is a powerful chemical change within the body that can literally be tasted in deep meditation. Soma is the sap of plants and tree. It is the "sap" of the human body, which is plasma.

An excellent mantra to Soma is:

Om Somaya Namaḥ.

Indra. Indra is the highest function of the mind. He is the cosmic person. He is the ruling power of our physical being.

An excellent mantra is Indra is:

Om Īm Indraya Namaḥ.

Surya. Surya is our soul essence, the sun. The sun is a daily reminder that our true essence is soul and light. Mantras and visualizations on Surya are to tap into our soul energies and consciousness.

Om Śum Suryaya Namaḥ.

These should be learned from a qualified teacher.

Goals of Vedic Yoga

As with all yoga systems, people may have numerous reasons for practicing Vedic yoga. Self-realization should be at the top of the list. Vedic yoga is an advanced, scientific, and powerful system for personal and planetary transformation. It is reasonable to assume that some preparation should be considered in the journey toward self-realization. As an example, it is reasonable that an individual would need to strengthen their mind and body; additionally, they would need to detoxify and purify their mind and body, as well. They would need preparation on an emotional and mental level, as the process of self-realization is often a radical shift within an individual's perception of reality. The process toward self-realization is beautifully illustrated in the Vedic battle between Indra and Vrtra.

Indra and Vrtra's battle

Within the Vedas is an important story relating to Indra and Vrtra. In later Hinduism, Indra is little more than a Deity of the rains or storms. While Indra and his thunderbolt can be associated with storms, in Vedic times Indra was considered the God of gods. While this may have little relevance to the western reader, Indra can be brought into light for the western mind. Indra is our true essence or being. Some might use the term soul, or the power of the soul.

Vrtra is often referred to as the adversary of Indra. Vrtra is also referred to as the dragon or serpent, which holds back the waters. These waters are released when Indra slays Vrtra.

Again, this can initially have little relevance to the western reader; however, Vrtra can be easily brought into light for the western mind. To understand Vrtra, one must first look to the root that forms the word: *Vr.*

Vr literally means, "to cover". It is interesting to note that *Vr* is also a name for Indra. In the Vedic system, Vrtra is a shadow of Indra; and some consider him the brother of Indra. So does this literally mean that Indra has slain his brother? Is this an earlier version of the Cain and Able story recorded in the Christian Bible? Most likely it is not. Vrtra is a reflection of Indra. This reflection covers and obscures our view of the true reality of nature. Just as a mountain can be reflected in a lake, the lake cannot be the mountain but only a reflection of it, a reflection (within the lake) that is easily disturbed. So what is this reflection that appears so pure and perfect?

This reflection would be called Vrtra, and Vrtra is a reference to the ego. More correctly, the ego is the concealing power of Vrtra. This power of Vrtra is referred to as "*Avarana Shakti*". Avarana Shakti can literally mean "the power to hinder in time and space." Vrtra is the root power of the ego, and has the power to hinder our spiritual growth in the field of time and space, but not the power to hinder our true power or essence (Indra). It would be correct to call it the root power of the ego. Vrtra later appears in Hindu philosophy as avidya (ignorance). It would also be correct to say that Vrtra is the power of maya in the world.

References to Indra slaying the serpent and releasing the waters are a teaching of spiritual realization; the cover of avidya (ignorance) being removed opening us to awareness of our true nature. This is the journey of humankind. Each individual consciously or unconsciously is traveling this path. This was clearly understood by the great rishis of the Vedic period. Their great gift to future generations was recorded in the Vedas and has been preserved for over 8500 years. While some scholars could argue that Indra's slaying of the serpent can also be a reference to awakening the Kundalini energy;

this should not be seen as a conflict with the underlying essence of Indra and Vrtra. It is more of an extension or other aspect of the Universal truth presented with Indra and Vrtra. It would also be correct to say that Vrtra is the Kundalini in a dormant (tamasic) state. Vrtra is the inertia that keeps the Kundalini from rising up the sushumna.

From the standpoint of chakras, Vrtra manifests as the lower manifestation of the manipura (3rd or navel) chakra. Actually, the lower functions of the first three chakras are the playground of Vrtra. In our society, it has been taught, at times, that the mind is ruled by the manipura chakra. Actually, our goal should be that the mind is ruled by the anahata chakra (4th or heart center). Once the minds activities are ruled or governed by the anahata chakra, the higher function of manipura chakra is activated, opening the power of *iccha shakti* (the power of the will, desire, and love). Iccha shakti should manifest through the power of the third chakra but directed by the higher functions of the anahata chakra. Indra's journey of slaying Vrtra really begins with meditation on the heart chakra, more correctly, on the spiritual heart chakra located within the field of the anahata chakra. One could also perform meditation on a flame within the heart center. The flame should be the size of the thumb. Initially, this should only be practiced for about 3 minutes.

Vrtra's Manifestation in the Physical Realm

Earlier we explored various attributes and qualities of Vrtra, especially the connection between the ego and Vrtra. One of the most important and overlooked attributes is the physical manifestation of Vrtra. Aside from the physical manifestations of the ego and the plethora of problematic manifestations this can cause, neglect of the literal physical manifestations can have dire consequences.

While there are numerous Vedic references to Vrtra being a cloud, serpent, demon, etc. as we have examined earlier; these can be references to qualities of mind. Even Yaska and his naturalistic interpretation in *The Nighantu and The Nirkuta* acknowledge that he is a demon, while this is not a demon as in the Christian view; it is a demon as in our lower negative thoughts; though in the naturalistic view it is a cloud. Within the same book there is a reference that the serpent (Vrtra) blocked the rivers by expanding his body, indicating a large ego, so to speak. And Indra's slaying of Vrtra results in the rivers opening. This has been explained in earlier sections. But what have not been explored are the physical manifestations of the blocked rivers.

From a purely physical standpoint one obvious example would be coronary heart disease. Initially this may appear a little strange, but in reality it makes perfect sense. The literal blockage is a perfect manifestation of the "serpent expanding its body and blocking the rivers." A closer examination of this concept reveals the body's link with the mental state of individual, and connection between the ego's grasp on our thoughts and their manifestation within the physical body. From this standpoint Vrtra is the temporary master or overlord of the body. This often results in Vrtra influencing the choices and decisions that we make in daily life; resulting in suffering. The journey of spirituality is one of obtaining freedom from the demonic overlord (Vrtra) and embracing our true essence (Indra).

The Vedic Vrtra: Ancient Term for the Ego

As stated earlier, society has often lost respect for ancient traditions, assuming that ancient peoples were ignorant, unsophisticated, and of a lower mentality. Yet, scientists suggest that the brain of the human animal has evolved little in the last 100,000 years. If this is true, then clearly ancient man had the same intellectual prowess as modern man.

To explore this concept, let's examine in more depth the ancient Vedic adversary known as Vrtra. Vrtra can represent numerous different principles and ideas within the spiritual world and world of matter, as we previously discussed. Vrtra is known as the shadow of Indra, the supreme mind. As Indra represents the higher mind, Vrtra represents the lower; which in and of itself can represent the ego, as the lower function of mind, from a spiritual standpoint. But there is a more interesting name for Vrtra that illustrates this even better, and it is known as "ahi".

The name Ahi occurs numerous times in the Vedas; particularly in reference to the destruction of ahi. The term "Ahi" is interesting as it refers to numerous qualities as does most Sanskrit terms. Ahi literally means: killing, a wicked man, a cheat, the sun, the planet Rahu, Vrtra, the aslesha nakshatra, a serpent or snake. Examining each of these terms reveals a clear reference to the ego.

The ego is viewed as killing, as it is the primary motivator of misery and suffering within the human condition. The ancient view of the ego was a wicked man and cheat, as it kept itself from the realization of the true essence of its own existence — soul.

From an astrological standpoint, the sun, in its lower manifestation represents the ego, as does the planet Rahu. Rahu is the north node of the moon, and represents the ego's tendency to gravitate towards issues of mass consciousness, or worldly consciousness. Rahu can also cause the mind to become easily influenced by lower negative tendencies. The ancient mind also viewed this as a function of the ego. The nakshatra (star) known as aslesha is interesting as it represents the serpent. In its higher manifestation, it is strongly associated with the Kundalini energy, and in its lower manifestation the ego. This is represented by the shakti (power) associated with ashlesha called *visasleshana shakti*, which is the power to inflict poison. The word "ahi" like the word "ahamkara" from the Samkhya philosophy represents the entire Sanskrit alphabet between its two letters (*ah* and *ha* giving aham which means I). The letters represent the numerous facets of our being, which in their lower manifestation comprise the ego.

It becomes clear that the ancient people had a clear concept of ego. A term that was not rediscoverd by modern science until the early 1900's. Yet, it is clearly defined, in different terms, from at least 6500 BCE by ancient man. Again, it appears that ancient societies, though less technical than modern society, had keen insight into the inner workings of our being.

The following list is a variety of techniques to begin the journey of your personal battle with Vrtra. The list is not comprehensive but is intended to provide several options for the Vedic yoga beginner to intermediate level student. Several of the techniques are best practiced under the guidance of a qualified Vedic or yoga teacher. Some of the techniques are of minor consideration but illustrate that anyone can practice regardless of their physical ability.

Beginning techniques for your personal (Indra) victory over Vrtra:

- Study of sacred scriptures such as the Vedas, Upanishads, or Vedantic philosophy. There are many excellent systems in India that can fulfill this need. Systems such as Karma or Bhakti yoga are important and serve as an important beginning to this journey.
- Almost any classical yoga system can aid in beginning the journey for Indra's victory over Vrtra. In fact, this is a major goal in true yoga systems, to strengthen the body, remove toxins and transform the ego. This is especially true of some Tantric systems, which seek to elevate and transform the ego. Or as Patanjali said so well: the seen perceives the seer.
- A yogic technique known, as flexion of the spine can be beneficial, as-well-as Bhastrika, often referred to as fire breathing or breath of fire. These techniques can easily be learned from a knowledgeable yoga teacher. They can also be found in several yoga/meditation books. They are contraindicated for pregnancy and various physical

limitations. Both of these techniques help to clear the sushumna especially the psychic knots (*granths*) in the sushumna. In yoga philosophy, these psychic knots must be cleared for spiritual realization to take place. In addition, they both generate tapas, which is a psychic heat that helps to purify the mind/body field.

- Pranayama exercises. Yogic breathing exercises teach the student to gain control over the mind. This eventually leads in the ability to go beyond mind. As yoga will teach us to go beyond body, pranayama is an important first step in the journey to go beyond the mind.
- Meditation is the most important and powerful tool for slaying Vrtra. It is interesting to note, in modern society people meditate to relax, while true meditation cannot occur until one is relaxed. The meditation I am referring to is not relaxation techniques, but deep inquiry into the nature of the self. However relaxation exercises can be an important first step for the beginner.
- Mula Bhanda. The *mula bhanda* (root lock) is a technique used to purify the sushumna (on a physical level the spinal column). It also helps to open the psychic knots of the sushumna. This technique should be practiced under the guidance of a teacher proficient in the practice of chakra locks, and caution is advised with this technique.
- Meditation on Vedic Deities. This serves to awaken us more to the Mahat (cosmic intelligence), moving our conscious mind beyond the ego. The deities are visualized with different colors and attributes depending on the need of each person.
- Meditating with the thumbs crossed. This is a common posture. Sitting crossed-legged, interlace the fingers with thumbs crossing over each other and resting in the webbing of the opposite hand. For males the right thumb should be crossed over the left. For females the left thumb should be crossed over the right. This adds a polarity

aspect to the mudra. This is a minor consideration, but does illustrate that everyone can work on Vrtra.

- Chanting the Sanskrit alphabet, or chanting the vowels of the Sanskrit alphabet. Indra rules the vowels of the Sanskrit alphabet.
- Chanting to Ganesh using the Bija mantra such as Om Gam Om.
- People that are astrologically oriented could use mantras such as Om hrīm brhaspataye namaḥ, but it is wise to consult a Vedic astrologer first.
- The bija mantra for Maha Maya. In some tantric systems, it is believed that only maha maya can provide a doorway from the covering of illusion (maya). Her bija mantra is Hrīm.
- Of course, the Rig Veda 1.10.5 gives insight into how to increase our Indra or ego defeating energy. It says in the first line: *Uktham indrāya śasyam vardhanam puruniṣṣdhe...*

Offer praise to Indra [with] hymns [mantra].

There are numerous riks (hymns) to Indra; these are best learned from a qualified Vedic yoga teacher.

- Performance or attendance of Homas, Pujas, or Yajnas. Homas are fire ceremonies, as can be yajnas. Pujas can be various internal and external forms of worship. This subject alone can be quite extensive; literally volumes of books have been written on these subjects. It does bring ritual to the practitioner's life, which can have a calming effect on the mind.

All afore mentioned techniques are part of the Vedic yoga system. But occasionally one may ask, "Why should I practice this form of yoga versus another form?" For the majority of yoga practitioners, the other forms of yoga should be practiced first. As the other common yoga systems provide initial purification and balancing of the mind and body, this process prepares a student for the practice of Vedic yoga. It is a rare and smaller number of students that move directly into Vedic yoga; as the practice of Vedic yoga requires a focused mind, which has been purified and balanced with asana (postures), Pranayama (breathing exercises), mantra, and meditation.

For most students of meditation, very little attention is given to purification of the mind and body. While this need for purification appears commonly in almost every ancient tradition, it has been given little value in the last hundred years or so. This critical component is an essential part of all yoga traditions, and especially Vedic yoga.

As an example, I chanted this mantra for years in preparation for the practice of Vedic yoga:

Punantu mā devajanaḥ
Punantu manavo dhiyā
Punantu viśva bhūtāni pavamānaḥ
Punātu mā

Atharva Veda B.6 H.19 v.1

Translation: "May the Gods (Divinity) purify me. May minds of knowledge purify me. May all universal minds purify me, may the poisons be removed."

This gentle purification was an essential component for preparing me for the more advanced states of Vedic yoga. Within this ancient system there is a simple formula to follow:

1) Study and practice leading to the TRUE realization with one's personal deity.

2) TRUE realization of the deity's oneness with Brahman (one consciousness or deity.)

So on one level the goals are preparation, purification, and strengthening of the body's subtle and physical systems. Additionally, it would be correct to say that Vedic yoga, in some instances, is an attempt to modify karma. From an eastern viewpoint all such systems are an attempt to modify karma. Vedic astrology (Jyotish) is a process and technology to understand and read karma. The remedial measures of Vedic astrology are an attempt to modify the karma. Ayurveda is an attempt to modify karma. Allopathic medicine is an attempt to modify karma. So the Vedic rituals and practices can be used as a tool to attempt to modify karma.

Beginning Vedic Yoga at Home

The following is a list of suggested meditations for the next step of Vedic yoga practice. Care should be used with these techniques, as they can be quite powerful, and one should have practiced the previous techniques for the suggested time prior to beginning this program. All times are the maximum times, and initially they should be started with considerable less time than the times or repetitions listed.

Usually, the first deity to start with in the Vedic system is Agni; though earlier we introduced Ushas due to the need to begin to enhance the spiritual awakening process. Within the Rig Veda the first mantra is to Agni. Within the Yajna system the first deity evoked is Agni. The following is a healing Yajna that is excellent for practitioners of Ayurveda as well as Vedic Yoga.

Meditation — on Agni Level 2 Agni Technique

1. Visualize a flame in the heart, or spiritual heart. Initially, this should be practiced for a maximum of 3 minutes. Increase slowly over time, slowly building to 108 repetitions. Then proceed to step two.
2. Chant *Om ram agnaye namaḥ*, while visualizing the flame becoming larger with each repetition. By the 54th repetition, the flame should surround the entire body. Once one is comfortable with this process, and having practiced for a considerable period of time, continue to step three.
3. Perform an offering of mantra into the flame of the 5 Vedantic prana mantras:

Om Prāṇaya Svaheti
Om Apānaya Svaheti
Om Samānaya Svaheti
Om Udānaya Svaheti
Om Vyānaya Svaheti

Continue to visualize the flame, and begin repetition of the mantra "Om Ram Agnaye Namaḥ", as the mantra is repeated the flame starts to become smaller and is brought into the root (muladhara) chakra. This image is held there. Continue until 54 repetitions of the mantra are completed.

Prana Offering Mantra

Om Prāṇaya Svaheti
Om Apānaya Svaheti
Om Samānaya Svaheti
Om Udānaya Svaheti
Om Vyānaya Svaheti

Another technique for balancing the vital energies is working with the different forms of prana or life-force energy. The key is that each line should be repeated for the same number of repetitions. Variations in repetitions could result in deranging the pranas. To practice this technique repeat line 1 a specific number of times, as an example twenty-seven times, then repeat line 2 twenty-seven times. Repeat this process until the last line has been completed. Any number can be used especially sacred numbers such as 54 or 108.

Note:

For level 1 (beginners) students repeat mantra aloud.

For level 2 (intermediate) students repeat ½ of the mantra repetitions aloud, ½ at a whisper.

This represents the Vedic fire ritual and performs to offerings into the fire, one speech (body), the other mind (whisper).

It is also good the chant each line, of the prana offering, once over food, prior to eating.

Outer Yajna
Short Ganash Puja

1-Chant the Purification Mantra (Punantu mantra).

2-Light ghee lamp.

3- Mentally ask Ganesh for help in removing obstacles to my study and spiritual growth.

4- Chant the Om Gam Gaṇapataye Namaḥ mantra 108 times.

5- Offer flower to feet of Ganesh, carnation any color for now.

Technique — Healing the Heart

Sitting crossed-legged, take the left hand and make the fingers even. Place the four fingers in a straight line (up and down) at the center of the chest.

Chant: Om Hrīm

Practice time 3 minutes.

5 Basic Yajnas

A very common Yajna practiced in India is the panchayajna. The five basic yajnas are:

1. Brahma Yajna — involves some form of daily study.
2. Deva Yajna — Mantra to a deity.
3. Pitra Yajna — One stick of incense — Om Hrīm Pitr Ya Namaḥ Feel that you are offering the incense to your ancestors.
4. Bhuta Yajna — Offering to nature, Incense, food offering with mantra Om Bhūta Ya Namaḥ.
5. Mimsa Yajna — Offerings to friends. Merely light incense with intention that it is an offering to friends and visitors.

These are important yajnas that almost anyone can do. The first is daily study. The deva yajna is mantras to various deities or deity of one's choice. The pitra yajna is an offering to our ancestors. After all, this body we have is the result of our karmas and all the actions performed by our ancestors. Bhuta is an offering to nature. And the Mimsa yajna is giving of food, drink etc to guests.

For many beginners this is probably the most important yajna to perform. It returns us to a realization of the sacredness of life and action. **In many ways this should be the yajna that everyone starts with!**

Additional Important Deities within the Vedic System

Vayu: An Introduction to the Divine Wind

The Vedic deity Vayu, is not a common term within modern society, but is one of the most important deities, especially pertaining to health and manifestation of the physical body.

The Sanskrit root to Vayu is *vaa* which means to "blow" or "to move". Vayu would be one of the first movements from the soul, (Purusha, paratman, Surya, Brahman), which is often referred to as prana. Within the Purusha (soul), Vayu exists as unmanifested power or consciousness. Within the realm of nature, Vayu manifests as Prana. Vayu manifesting as prana is responsible for the manifestation of all creation.

Vayu manifests as prana and its subtle forms called:

1. Udana — Our creative expression, upward moving spirituality.
2. Apana — The manifesting current into the world. Elimination and detoxification.
3. Samana — The equalizing force of the universe.
4. Vyana —The outward circulating force of the universe.
5. Prana — the vital force of all creation.

From a yogic standpoint, Prana and Apana are the most important, as they represent vitality and elimination of toxins. From a cosmic standpoint, Prana starts the cycle of creation by moving from a sattvic (harmonious) state into a Rajasic (active) state. Apana gives firmness to the creation or form, by providing downward movement for manifestation. The form (matter) is maintained by the constant influx of new energy and the removal of old (prana and apana).

On a quantum level, energy is in constant movement even though it may appear stationary to the eye. As an example, looking at a wall, it appears as solid matter. In reality, it is a vibrating mass of energy in constant movement. It appears solid only because the molecules in our body are dense enough to not be able to pass through the wall. In the case of water, though there is still density of molecules, they are not dense enough to obstruct the body from passing through them. The same principle applies to air which is even less in density.

Samana provides stability between the inflow and outflow of energy, providing stabilization. Vyana provides the outer flow of energy for more manifestation, or the circulating flow throughout the field of manifestation. Udana provides upward flow or movement toward a more primal state of being. Primal is not to imply a lower or lesser-evolved state in this case. This same process can be applied to all levels of creation, including the human body.

This process is evidenced within the universe, the solar system, the physical body, and even on the cellular level. As an example, on the cellular level, Prana is the vital air coming to the cell via the blood. Apana is the release of carbon, wastes, and other materials from the cell back into the blood stream. Samana is the balance between these two forces (prana and apana) within the cell. Udana is the higher function of the cell for the health of the body; it is also the communication between cells via chemical messengers. Vyana is the circulation of the vital force throughout the cell.

According to Pandit Vamadeva Shastri (David Frawley), Vayu is also known as *sutratman*. Sutratman consists of two words: Sutra (thread) and Atman, literally meaning the soul's threads. This is reference to the nadis of the astral and physical body, clearly indicating that Vayu is responsible for the flow of energy (prana) through the body's nadis. With this understanding, Vayu becomes the lord of all life, nervous energy, and movement.

Vayu in the Vedas

Within the Rig Veda, Vayu, at times, is included in hymns with Indra (the higher mind). A more modern day example from India would be Shiva and Shakti. The argument arises, who is more important Shiva (Divine consciousness) or Shakti (Divine Power). While different philosophical systems answer this differently, I would like to suggest that both are equally important. Divine power needs Divine consciousness guiding it. Likewise, Divine consciousness is impotent without Divine power to manifest its will; therefore, both are equally important. Certainly this is true within the Vedic system, where Vayu the divine manifesting power is similar to Shakti though not viewed as a feminine force. The relationship between Indra and Vayu represents this same line of thought. On a personal level, Indra represents the mental principle, or mental ability and Vayu represents the manifestation of the principle and the vital energy flowing through the body. From this standpoint, it is clear why they would be included in suktas (hymns) together on occasions, as they do within the Rig Veda on occasion.

Other deities are often invoked for the pranas and their healing ability; within the Vedas most commonly we find references to horses or the Ashvins. It is important to note that the Ashvins are horses and associated with Ushas. In this function, they are representing the transition from darkness (ignorance) to light (knowledge). They are considered the twin physicians also. This is a clear indication of their association with prana/Vayu. This is not in contradiction, but is most likely an expression of a power of Vayu. ***The Nirukta***, a classic text confirms this, "They are three gods: Agni in earth, Vayu or Indra in atmosphere and Surya in heaven. Each of them is known by various names depending on the different actions performed."(1) As mentioned earlier, the Ashvins are Prana and Apana on one level, though they would not be limited to this function alone. They are not to be contradictory to Vayu but are additional expressions and expansions of this energy, as stated above in ***The Nirukta***.

The horse is a common symbol used in the Vedas to represent the stamina and power of prana. Indra has steeds as-well-as Surya. Indicating their power (shakti) via Vayu. Vayu has steeds called *niyut*, which means to unite. Vayu (prana) unites the three Vedic worlds called Prithivi (Earth), Antariksha (Atmosphere), and Dyau (Heaven); meaning that prana unites these worlds. Vayu is the ruler of the middle world Antariksha (atmosphere). In Vedic cosmology, antariksha is considered the most important world as it separated the earth and the heavens, giving birth to creation. Examples of other deities associated with the atmosphere (antariksha) are Indra and Shiva.

Vayu is an important Vedic deity for understanding the unfolding universe and our physical manifestation. While more importance is placed on Surya, Indra and certainly Agni, Vayu's importance cannot be underestimated. When mantra combining Indra and Vayu is applied, a potent force is awakened within the conscious being for health, and spiritual awareness. Vayu represents our awakening to the potential of the mind and its power. The primary expression is prana, but Vayu represents so many different levels of power, force, and the energy of consciousness.

Vayu is a drinker of soma within the Vedic system; in fact all the deities drink soma. Soma has numerous meanings, but in the context of this book, Vayu drinks the vitality of the sensory impressions. This in turn feeds and vitalizes the pranas of the mind and body. This makes sensory impressions a form of soma or food for Vayu. It determines the quality of prana within the mind and body. Once clearly understood, the vital link between yoga and the Vedic teachings becomes quite clear.

Vayu, Yoga and Ayurveda

The relationship between Vayu and yoga cannot be denied, once the connection between Vayu and prana is established. Prana can be increased through a variety of tools, especially Vedic mantras to Vayu. Pranayama is just another expression of the worship of Vayu. While terms such as worship are often upsetting to western students, the act of breathing should be an act of worship. It is a bhakti (devotional) act that is performed tens of thousands of times each day. Each breath can be a silent mantra to Vayu. Each breath can be a silent affirmation of the pulsating energy from the cosmic mind. Tapas or psychic heat is generated by pranayama (Vayu).

Just these few examples clearly illustrate the relationship between yoga and Vayu. Without the vital air there would be no creation, existence, or life. In addition, Vayu has an important link with Ayurveda. As one important attribute of Ayurveda is "Pranic Healing", Vayu's role as a healer becomes apparent, though it was often expressed in later Vedic times with the Ashvins. Without the energy of prana, the fire of Tejas cannot burn brightly. Without Tejas the mind becomes weak, clouded, and slow in function. Vayu flows through the Nadi's and marmas for healthy energy within the body's subtle energy system, the chakra system, and the physical organs themselves. Vata is the subtle biological manifestation of Vayu. One aspect of Ayurvedic rejuvenation therapy is increasing/balancing prana within the body. This is illustrated with herbs such as ashwangdha and bala. Triphala increases the colon's ability to eliminate toxins, balancing high vata in the colon and increasing the body's vitality and ability to detoxify.

Vayu plays an important role within the physical body. It is also present within the mental or emotional bodies. The importance of the 5 major forms of prana cannot be underestimated, and Vayu is the ruling deity behind them[1].

---

[1]Roy, Raja Ram Mohan "Vedic Physics" 1999 Canada: Golden Egg Publishing.

An Introduction to Sarasvati

Sarasvati ancient goddess of the Vedas, she has existed before recorded time, but what does she mean and how does she relate to the modern student of spirituality?

As with most terms within Sanskrit, the meaning and usage of a word has changed dramatically over time. Initially, western scholars doubted the existence of the Vedic river named Sarasvati; eventually reducing it to a river in Afghanistan or the Indus river. Recent archaeological discoverers have clearly demonstrated the location of the Sarasvati river, and the discovery of cities and towns along its banks, clearly demonstrating that the Sarasvati river was not a myth but a reality.

The literal Sarasvati River was a river flowing from the receding glaciers of the last Ice Age to the ocean. Satellite analysis suggests that the river was of tremendous size; and writings within the Vedas illustrate that it played a vital role within the life and spiritual life of the Vedic people along its banks.

The word Sarasvati comes from the word *sare*, which means fluid or liquid. Sara comes from the verbal root *Sr* meaning "to flow". Due to the different schools that developed within the Vedic teachings, this meaning was extended into a variety of areas. Within Ayurveda (an upaveda — secondary Vedas), Sarasvati is also a nadi running from the tailbone to the tip of the tongue, which explains Sarasvati's strong connection with speech in later Hindu teachings. So it would be correct to perform mantra to Sarasvati to strengthen or help with speech. It would also be correct to say that Sarasvati is the proper flow or rhythm of the Vedic mantras themselves. She also represents the flow of life through the body via prana and the circulatory system.

In the earlier Vedic period, Sarasvati was most commonly associated with inspiration. Likewise, it would be correct to perform mantra to Sarasvati for inspiration. This same concept is reflected in the later teachings within Hinduism from the Puranas, but Sarasvati is replaced with Ganga as portions of the Vedic culture had moved to the Gangic region as the Sarasvati dried up approximately 1900 BCE. Within the puranas, Sarasvati is a manifestation of Shakti, or the feminine power. So mantras to Sarasvati are mantras to Shakti as well.

Mantras to Sarasvati help to cultivate fluidity and flowing movement within our lives. Providing the ability to flow with obstacles and challenges rather than bashing against them. Being the most sacred of the seven Vedic rivers, she is the primal flow that energizes the 7 chakras of the astral body.

Mantra to Sarasvati can bestow learning, and prosperity to the aspirant. She is strongly associated with the Gods and Manu (which can be a reference to the mind). As the consort of Manu (mind), Sarasvati is the prosperous flow of energy from the mind. She is also associated with the waters being released with Indra's victory over Vrtra (Soul over Ego).

There are numerous mantras to Sarasvati within the Vedas, but for most western students it would be easiest to begin with simple bija mantras such as "Aim". Mantras such as "Om Aim" are excellent to start with. This mantra is especially good for students and situations involving learning.

Bhakti

Bhakti (devotion) was discussed earlier in relation to the *Yoga Sutras of Patanjali*, but bhakti is also an important part of yoga and especially Vedic yoga. The role of bhakti is often downplayed in our modern world. Science has caused us to move away from devotion, and we often look to science to explain all things. Science has an important role in the world. Likewise, it is not realistic to expect science to explain everything, as science is evolving in its own right. In terms of yoga practice, clearly bhakti yoga has more practitioners than any other system globally.

Bhakti is an important part of Vedic yoga. Like all spiritual systems, it has its literalist and its abstract thinkers. Each serves a vital role in growing spirituality within the individual. Some scholars suggest that bhakti is antiquated and does not really belong in the modern "scientific" age. But bhakti plays many important roles, especially in the realm of transformation of the ego. As the ego begins to become transformed, bhakti helps the ego to recognize that there is something greater than it, allowing the ego to move beyond the self centered position that it usually occupies. Through bhakti and within the field of the ego, arises a desire to know this greater essence — devatas. By recognizing the role, or many roles, that the devatas play, the ego is slowly elevated and transformed; rather than being destroyed — the ego is transformed or more correctly merged with its true essence — soul, atman, Purusha.

Bhakti also opens our heart. As our heart opens, we become more open to the possibilities of spiritual realization. It is our personal spiritual realization through our relationship with the devatas that we are transformed, or more correctly realize our true nature or essence. This transformation allows us to transcend the daily challenges of life. This is not to imply that we can avoid all challenges of life, but rather we deal with them differently. A harmony and flow begins to develop and evolve within each of us, though the grace of the divine energies that flow forth from Brahman and manifest as the devatas. Many of the slokas (hymns) in the Vedas have a bhakti element to them. So it is important to cultivate the devotional aspect within our yoga practice. Here are some examples of ways to cultivate bhakti:

- Spending time with spiritual people.
- Visiting spiritual places.
- Cultivating spiritual desire and devotion within our hearts.
- Study of spiritual teachings or scriptures.
- Singing of bhajans is beneficial.
- Chanting mantra is one of the most effective ways to cultivate bhakti.
- Meditation at temples.
- Performing traktek on deities.
- Visualization of images of a deity.
- Creating a sacred space in the home for an altar.
- Creating a space for meditation in the home.
- Cultivating a relationship with a teacher, acharya or Guru.
- Approaching all activities with a sense of reverence.
- Daily meditation.

Vedic Deities and Yoga in Western Culture

Is there any Relevance to the Modern Western Practitioner?

While yoga has been growing within western culture for almost one hundred years, within the United States, one can observe a tremendous surge in popularity since the sixties, to the most recent indicators suggesting that millions of Americans now practice yoga in some form or another.

While the roots of yoga are most certainly linked with and a part of Hinduism and its most important teachings known as the Vedas, or books of knowledge, the average yoga student has little exposure or awareness of the ancient roots to yoga. While many students are looking to escape religion, or certainly not looking for a new religion; for many, at best, they are open to new age spirituality. While this new type of spirituality borrows heavily from many of the great eastern traditions such as Hinduism, it is rare that they offer a comprehensive system of study. Often deities are relegated to a backseat within the new age philosophical model. The result has been a lessening of the understanding of deities, and the important role they play within spiritual growth. The ultimate result being that this is becoming a world devoid of conscious understanding regarding deities. What are the place, role and relevance for these Vedic deities? Their timeless wisdom, spanning eternity, as recorded in the Vedas. Or are they to become forgotten myths from some distant ancient people. Will their relevance with yoga become an abandoned teaching, or are they waiting for each student to discover their secret meanings?

To explore this, a westerner must learn to look at eastern teachings through eastern eyes. The literalist tradition, common in the west and relevant in the east, does not afford much opportunity to unlock the vast secrets held within the eastern traditions and the more familiar system of yoga. Western scholars tell us that yoga is one of 6 distinct traditions from the Indian subcontinent. But in reality, these traditions were intended to blend, to cross the lines of demarcation so frequently used in scholarly circles. The main 6 traditions are in reality a part of much greater whole, which afforded different approaches to the same truth. The separation of these systems has led to a decline in understanding and application of these powerful systems. This has resulted in deities being given a "backseat" role in many yoga centers. Often the western student wishes to merely confine deities to the realm of religion, whereas the eastern student and mystic realizes that the deities "blur" the lines to reality, and manifest in a variety of forms, and applications.

As an example, the Vedic deity Ushas literally means the dawn. But Ushas also symbolizes each person's awakening to truth. Ushas is the principle operating each time we connect, realize, or gain some insight into our life. With this understanding of Ushas it becomes difficult to say that Ushas is not relevant. In reality, Ushas has a significant role within each person's life, especially if they are oriented toward any type of personal growth or understanding. The Vedic battle between Indra and Vrtra, merely represents the battle between our higher and lower nature. Or some would say our spirit (soul) and ego. Both of these examples have relevance for most students of yoga. But as these teachings come from a different culture, we are often not familiar with the terms or we struggle with its symbolic representations. To deepen one's understanding of this process I will use the following story:

Within Indian legend there was a story of a great sage named Vasishtha. He owned a cow named Nandini, who was trapped in a huge gorge. The sage appealed to Lord Shiva, and

Shiva sent Sarasvati to flood the gorge so the cow could float free. For many students of yoga, this story has little relevance, unless one understands the symbolism behind the story. The cow being trapped represents blocked knowledge. Shiva represents higher knowledge. Sarasvati represents inspiration. The release of the cow is the opened flow of knowledge through higher inspiration. While this is a simplistic view of the story, it does illustrate the deeper meaning. Literally, an article could be written on the symbology of this story alone. While there could be numerous additional interpretations of this legend, the point I am trying to make is that we all have moments when creativity, or knowledge has difficulty flowing. We often seek inspiration to unlock the inner resources of the mind. Again these deities represent common cosmic principles and represent not just the mystical, but also the practical application of life principles. As the deities represent universal truths, they have universal application that transcends social and cultural differences. This view and way of looking at the world repeats itself frequently within the yoga tradition.

As the ancient yoga practitioners realized that the world was divine and a reflection of higher principles and truth. They would have been known as Animist. Not the animist of western scholars. Regrettably, the scholarly view of animism often portrayed ancient people as easily frightened by the sun, moon, night, and other common events. The true animists realized the divinity of life. They knew that each part played a role in the greater whole. They named postures after animals; elements and higher principle's call deities. They recognized that deities represented physiological and psychological aspects of creation as well. They also knew that the deities represent higher principles, and/or principles of physics. As an example, modern physics recognized 3 states of matter:

1). Solid.
2). Liquid.
3). Gas.

These fundamental concepts are reflected in the chakra system within yoga. In this system, each chakra is associated with an element. These elements move from dense (solid or earth) to gas (ether and air). Within this ancient tradition we find the building blocks of modern day physics.

Within the ***Atharva Veda***, one can find teachings of modern day visualization and affirmation tools; with such quotes as, "My mind stands against disease." (Atharva Veda) Another insightful mantra from the *Yajur Veda* (Shukla version) is:

Preserve my life.
Assist/Preserve my prana (life-force).
Assist/preserve my vyana (circulating life-force).
Assist/preserve my sight.
Assist/preserve my ears [hearing].
Assist/preserve my speech, let it abound.
Be active in my mind.
Keep my soul.
[Keep] my light pure.
Yajur Veda XIV.17

This is a powerful affirmation for health and wellness.

Even electrical polarity was represented by the masculine and feminine principles. In fact, postures were divided into masculine and feminine postures based on their effect on the body and mind. Giving birth to the world's first polarity therapy, this appears within the Ayurvedic tradition. Postures were recognized as heating and cooling, as well; and an entire system of practice was developed around these very principles, as well. All of these qualities have deities associated with them, representing a system that has more depth and complexity than our modern periodic table. The deities are combined in various mantras, breathing exercises and postures, with the same sophistication and precision as the modern chemist mixes formulas.

They (Hindus) recognized that the senses offered food (sensory experience) to the mind. And that the senses had a powerful impact on the activities, desires, and attractions of the mind. But more importantly, they recognized that the different flows of consciousness emanated from more than just the mind. They realized that greater flows of consciousness flowed from the soul level and through the mind, ultimately looking to manifest on a physical level. These various flows of consciousness are Vedic deities.

A clear example of this is with the Vedic Deity Agni (fire). On a personal and physical level Agni is a very important teaching. As Agni manifests in the physical body as the digestive fire and metabolism, within Ayurveda this is called Jatharagni. There is also the fire of the mind, the ability to digest experience. This is also a form of Agni. So it is literally impossible to say that Agni is not important.

For modern day yoga practitioners, the oldest form of yoga we have in written form is "Vedic Yoga". Vedic yoga is filled with deities and their practical application on a multitude of levels, offering a variety of techniques depending on the consciousness and ability of the practitioner. While Vedic yoga does not contain the postures commonly associated with yoga. It does contain mudras (hand positions) for meditation, mantra, pranayama (breathing exercises), and meditation itself. Vedic yoga contains many of the elements that are common within other systems of yoga. It has information and references to the kundalini, which is represented by the kundalini yoga tradition. It has the sun and moon of the Hatha yoga tradition. It contains wisdom representing the Jnana yoga tradition. Certainly the Bhakti yoga tradition (Yoga of Devotion) is represented within the Vedas, and its reverence for the deities. Numerous traditions can trace their roots to the Vedas such as the Tantric yoga tradition and others. In fact, elements of "Vedic Yoga" appear within most of the ancient traditions from India. Ranging from texts such as the *Agamas*, *Tantras*, and even the "*Yoga Sutras of Patanjali*", which is probably one of the best-known texts for western students.

From the ancient perspective, the deities represent opportunities to transform the mind and body on a subtle and gross physical level, increasing harmony, peace, and overall wellness. They offer tools for dealing with negativity and practical counsel on living a productive life. For the modern day practitioner, these ancient deities afford a fast track for personal and planetary transformation. They awaken healing energies within the mind and body. They provide access into the deeper regions of the mind, resulting in expanding awareness and mental performance. But most importantly they offer the opportunity for spiritual transformation and realization. From the eastern viewpoint and especially the yoga traditions, it is impossible to separate yoga from the deities, as they represent the universal forces of creation and transformation.

Conclusion

While appearing new as far as modern publication is concerned, Vedic Yoga is not a new trend. In reality, it is the mother to all yoga systems. Vedic Yoga is the spiritual essence of all yoga systems. All classical yoga texts reference back to the teachings, deities, and principle's of the Vedas. Though terms may have changed over the millennia, the modern day practitioner has a rare opportunity to experience what was literally reserved for only a few practitioners of deep spirituality.

Through the patient application of the techniques in this book, a new world of spirituality, eternal truth and teachings will slowly start to open. This is the goal and purpose of yoga. To unite! To join our lower mind with the true essence of our higher reality and identity. Through the practice of Vedic Yoga, one begins to experience the essence of yoga. The key is patience, practice, and perseverance.

Bibliography

Aurobindo, Sri "The Secret of the Veda" Sri Aurobindo Ashram Trust: Pondicherry 1996

Beal, Yogi Baba Prem Tom "Understanding the Kundalini" Universal Yoga www.vedicpath.com

Beal, Yogi Baba Prem Tom "Qualities of a Student" www.vedicpath.com

Beal, Yogi Baba Prem Tom "Vrtra: The Spiritual Adversary" Vedic Friends Journal #1 http://www.vedicfriends.org vfa_journal_and_newsletter.htm

Beal, Yogi Baba Prem Tom "Introduction to the roots of the kundalini" Universal Yoga 2003

Beal, Yogi Baba Prem, "Introduction to the Yoga Sutras". Universal Yoga 2000.

Beal, Yogi Baba Prem, "Introduction to the Yoga Sutras". Universal Yoga 2000.

Feuerstein, George. "The Shambhala Encyclopedia of Yoga" Shambhala Publications:Boston 1997

Frawley, David "Gods, Sages and Kings" Passage Press: Salt Lake City 1991

Frawley, David "The Rig Veda and the History of India" Aditya:Nw Delhi 2001

Frawley, David "Wisdom of the Ancient Seers: mantras of the Rg Veda" Passage Press: Salt Lake City 1992

Frawley, David "Yoga and Ayurveda" Lotus Press: Twin Lakes: Wisconsin 1999

Frawley, David "The Rig Veda and the History of India" Aditya Prakashan:Delhi 2001

Frawley David & Prem, Yogi Baba "Meditations on the Sacred Fire" CD Universal Yoga

Kashyap, Dr. R.L "Rig Veda Samhita:First Ashtaka Vol. 1,2,3" Saksivc:Bangalore

Beal, Yogi Baba Prem, "Introduction to the Yoga Sutras". Universal Yoga 2000.

Roy, Raja Ram Mohan "Vedic Physics" 1999 Canada: Golden Egg Publishing.
Saraswathi, Swamit Ramananda "Tripura Rahasya" World Wisdom 2002
Varenne, Jean. 1989. Yoga and the Hindu Tradition. Translated from French by Derek Coltman. Delhi: Motilal Banarsidas, 253 pages.
Sanskrit Texts:
Vayu Purana
Vishnu Purana
Tripura Rahasya
The Nighantu and The Nirukta
Yoga Sutras of Patanjali
Rg Veda
Yajur Veda
Taittiriya Samhita of the Krishna Yajur Veda
Shatapatha Brahmana (Kanva)
Paramananda Tantra
Gautamiya Tantra
Shaktisangamatantra
AgamaKosha Vol. 5 Prof S.K. Ramachandra Rao
Mahabhasya
Nighantu and Nirukta
Krishna Yajur Veda, Taittiriya Samhita
Hatha Yoga Pradipika
Shiva Samhita
Bhagavad Gita
Atharva Veda
Shukla Yajur Veda
Satapathabrahmana (Kanva)
The Nighantu and The Nirukta

Recommended Webpages
www.vedicpath.com
www.vedanet.com

Index